Visit our website

to find out about other books from Churchill Livingstone
and our sister companies in Harcourt Health Sciences

Register free at
www.harcourt-international.com

and you will get

- the latest information on new books, journals and electronic products in your chosen subject areas

- the choice of e-mail or post alerts or both, w̶h̶e̶r̶e̶ there are any new books in your chose̶n̶ a̶r̶

- news of speci

- information abo̶u̶t̶ Sciences companies incl̶ t̶o̶ne, and Mosby

You will also fi̶n̶ ̶dering, information on ̶ore!

Visit the Ha̶r̶c̶ou̶r̶

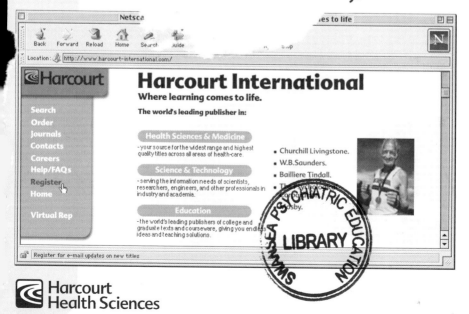

Netsca̶ ̶ ̶ ̶ ̶es to life

Back Forward Reload Home Search Guide

Location: http://www.harcourt-international.com/

Harcourt International
Where learning comes to life.

The world's leading publisher in:

Health Sciences & Medicine
- your source for the widest range and highest quality titles across all areas of health-care.

Science & Technology
- serving the information needs of scientists, researchers, engineers, and other professionals in industry and academia.

Education
- the world's leading publishers of college and graduate texts and courseware, giving you endless ideas and teaching solutions.

- Churchill Livingstone.
- W.B. Saunders.
- Bailliere Tindall.
- T̶h̶e̶ ̶ ̶ ̶
- ̶ ̶osby.

Search
Order
Journals
Contacts
Careers
Help/FAQs
Register
Home

Virtual Rep

Register for e-mail updates on new titles

Harcourt Health Sciences

Critical Appraisal
for Psychiatry

Commissioning Editor: Michael Parkinson
Project Development Manager: Siân Jarman
Design Direction: Erik Bigland
Project Manager: Nancy Arnott

Critical Appraisal for Psychiatry

Stephen M. Lawrie MD (Hons), MRCPsych, MPhil
Senior Clinical Research Fellow
Edinburgh University Department of Psychiatry
Royal Edinburgh Hospital, Edinburgh

Andrew M. McIntosh BSc (Hons), MB ChB, MRCPsych
Lecturer
Edinburgh University Department of Psychiatry
Royal Edinburgh Hospital, Edinburgh

Sanjay Rao MB BS, MD
Senior House Officer in Psychiatry
Royal Edinburgh Hospital, Edinburgh

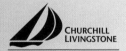

CHURCHILL
LIVINGSTONE

EDINBURGH LONDON NEW YORK PHILADELPHIA ST LOUIS
SYDNEY TORONTO 2000

CHURCHILL LIVINGSTONE
An imprint of Harcourt Publishers Limited

© Harcourt Publishers Limited 2000

 is a registered trademark of Harcourt Publishers Limited

The rights of S. M. Lawrie, A. M. McIntosh and S. Rao to be
identified as authors of this work have been asserted by them
in accordance with the Copyright, Designs and Patents Act
1988

First published 2000

ISBN 0 443 07017 2

British Library Cataloguing in Publication Data
A catalogue record for this book is available from the British
Library

Library of Congress Cataloging in Publication Data
A catalog record for this book is available from the Library of
Congress

Note
Medical knowledge is constantly changing. As new
information becomes available, changes in treatment,
procedures, equipment and the use of drugs become
necessary. The authors and the publishers have taken care to
ensure that the information given in this text is accurate and
up to date. However, readers are strongly advised to confirm
that the information, especially with regard to drug usage,
complies with the latest legislation and standards of practice.

Typeset by IMH(Cartrif), Loanhead, Scotland

Preface

This book is aimed primarily at psychiatric trainees sitting the MRCPsych part II. It should also appeal to more senior and junior psychiatrists, other mental health professionals and managers who need a relatively brief but comprehensive introduction to the underlying concepts and practice of evidence-based mental health (EBMH). It will be required reading for clinical tutors and for any psychiatrist who needs more than the haphazard insights gleaned from workshops and conferences.

Doctors (and perhaps especially psychiatrists) are generally ignorant about research methods, statistics and critical appraisal, but the recent drive towards evidence-based medicine and clinical governance means that all doctors will have to possess these skills. Being able to critically appraise clinical research is an essential part of modern medicine. This ability is enhanced by an understanding of the various research methods and statistical techniques, and is central to the implementation of evidence-based healthcare.

More cogently, the MRCPsych part II exam has, since 1999, included a critical appraisal paper. The Royal College of Psychiatrists has published a lengthy list of references, as an exam syllabus, but most trainees will not have the time or the inclination to read through them. General textbooks of psychiatry do not cover all the main topics in sufficient detail. Exam aids and books on evidence-based medicine are available but are either inadequate as a basic text or are aimed at a general medical readership. Until now there has been no single source for all the required information written specifically for a psychiatric audience.

This book runs through the principal components of research methods, relevant statistics and critical appraisal processes. We have based the text on the relevant parts of the 'subjects basic to psychiatry' for the MRCPsych in general (principles of evaluation and psychometrics, epidemiology and research) and the syllabus for the critical appraisal paper in particular. It is therefore detailed enough to attract those seeking a comprehensive introduction to the relevant areas, but short enough to be digestible. An everyday clinical relevance is maintained throughout, with examples from the psychiatric literature where possible.

The introductory chapter puts EBMH in a contemporary clinical context. The main part of the book then considers research methods, statistics and critical appraisal in that order. The critical appraisal checklists are derived from the work of David Sackett et al, for which acknowledgements are due. The next chapter provides some mock exam papers and model answers, designed for MRCPsych trainees but which should also be useful teaching aids for all readers. Finally, we include a glossary of definitions of key terms.

We have written this book to be read right through, but the critical appraisal chapter is sufficiently detailed to be self-contained. You may, none the less, benefit from obtaining the papers discussed in that chapter and reading them in tandem with the text, as we can only summarize the essential details here.

The combination of knowledge and experience gained from reading this book, and from attempting the multiple choice questions and mock exam papers, should help the average trainee to sail through the critical appraisal paper. More information is generally given than is required to pass the exam, but we think the detail facilitates understanding and hope that it will stimulate at least some readers to apply some of the techniques in their own research and clinical practice.

The relevant topics are covered to give the average practising clinician the skills to deal with what will be routinely expected as a result of the increasing drive towards evidence-based practice in mental health. When revalidation becomes part of a psychiatrist's continuing professional development, and a condition of continuing employment, it is very likely that all psychiatrists will have to demonstrate a working knowledge of what is described herein.

One thing is certain: trainees who find this book helps them to pass the MRCPsych part II will be able to use it as a reference resource for the foreseeable remainder of their professional lives.

Edinburgh   S.M.L.
2000   A.M.
       S.R.

Contents

5 Mock exam papers and model answers 189

1

Putting it all in context

Psychiatry and neurology only became distinct medical specialties about a century ago. The large psychiatric hospitals built by the Victorians were places of refuge (asylum) rather than treatment. Treatment of 'severe mental illness' became a political and medical priority when patient numbers showed no signs of abating. The widespread acceptance of 'neurosis' as legitimate illness, and psychotherapy as a treatment, can be attributed to the devastating effects of 'shellshock' during the First World War. Biomedical treatments were developed and often enthusiastically administered to patients, with varying rates of beneficial and adverse effects.

The efficacy of these treatments could not be rigorously evaluated until the 'invention' of the randomized controlled trial, the first reported use in medicine being an evaluation of streptomycin in treating tuberculosis by Bradford Hill in 1952. Antidepressants and antipsychotics were serendipitously discovered in the same decade, but were first evaluated in the 1960s. As the number of drugs available and evidence of their efficacy increased, the influence of psychoanalysis waned. The need for reliable ways of differentiating disorders that might respond to particular interventions required the development of operationalized diagnostic classification systems. None the less, Cochrane (1972) thought that psychiatry was still basically inefficient, primarily through a neglect of treatment appraisal (although he awarded his wooden spoon to obstetrics).

The recent history of psychiatric services is one of basically good ideas hindered by insufficient resources and inadequate evaluation. Community care is all too often manifest as neglect. Clinical audit and continuing medical education have also been ineffective.

1

Managers are often out of touch with clinical issues. Bureaucracy runs wild, swamping clinicians in the 'meetings culture'. The wider rise of a culture of narcissism and complaint has raised patients' expectations at precisely the time doctors are least able to meet them. Psychiatry is once more a respectable part of medicine, but the stigmatization of psychiatric disorders and patients remains a major problem. We have seen slow but steady gains in our understanding of the major psychiatric disorders. We have an ever-increasing array of drug and talking treatments of proven efficacy, but need to know what works best for whom. The evidence-based medicine movement, in its widest sense, appears to offer some solutions, but requires adequate support and has yet to demonstrate its own effectiveness.

What, then, can be sensibly predicted for the near future? Given adequate resources, the ideal psychiatric service in the foreseeable future might look something like this: the managers are clinicians; psychiatrists lead multidisciplinary teams in which everyone is encouraged to develop specific areas of expertise (e.g. substance abuse, psychotherapy); patient episodes are routinely recorded on a local computer database (as problems, interventions, outcomes) for individualized feedback and overall monitoring; the service is continually fine-tuned to ensure effectiveness, optimize outcomes and promote patient satisfaction; treatments are guided by evidence-based protocols, developed by local clinicians trained in critical appraisal, based upon national guidelines; a clinical governance officer coordinates these processes of staff development, audit and getting evidence into routine practice.

Many of these processes are already here or inevitable. There is a need for a book that describes critical appraisal in the context of a thoroughly modern evidence-based clinically governed service.

CLINICAL GOVERNANCE

Clinical governance can be defined as the means by which healthcare organizations ensure the provision of quality care by making individuals accountable for setting, maintaining and monitoring performance standards. It is a term coined by the current chief medical officer of England and Wales (Scally & Donaldson 1998) to encompass a number of related processes (Box 1.1).

Box 1.1   Key components of clinical governance

1. Quality improvement
2. Continuing professional development
3. Using scientific evidence to ensure clinical effectiveness
4. Promoting a culture of systematic evaluation
5. Risk reduction
6. Developing useful information systems

---

1. **Quality improvement** is the overall aim of clinical governance but depends on the other components being realized. It requires an explicit statement of standards to be met, as well as a monitoring system. Quality standards can include professional performance, the efficiency of resource use, risk management and patient satisfaction. Needs assessment, working with users/carers and qualitative studies are likely to be increasingly important in setting standards, but these will have to reflect attainable outcomes that are of interest to both clinicians and patients.

2. **Continuing professional development** (CPD) is achieved through individuals being facilitated to identify their training needs and monitor their progress in realizing them. This is likely to become part of revalidation. Note that CPD is distinct from continuing medical education, which simply does not improve the quality of healthcare (Davis et al 1995), but CPD has yet to demonstrate that it is an effective replacement.

3. **Using scientific evidence to ensure clinical effectiveness**. Clinical effectiveness is the extent to which an intervention (whether a treatment, a procedure or a service) improves the outcome for patients in clinical practice. It should be noted that randomized controlled trials measure efficacy, i.e. whether something works or not, whereas effectiveness – whether something works in clinical practice – is determined by pragmatic clinical trials and audit. A clinically effective service will make use of national and local guidelines, based on the results of audit and clinical trials, as clinical guidelines are able to improve health outcomes (Woolf et al 1999). The National Institute for Clinical Excellence (NICE) in England and Wales and the Scottish Health Technology Assessment Centre (SHTAC) and regional development and evaluation committees will be important in providing reliable clinical guidelines and in setting treatment priorities.

4. **Promoting a culture of systematic evaluation.** This includes audit and much more. Audit, along with community care,

was initially developed by doctors but suffered from being politically enforced and underfunded. There is no absolute distinction between audit and clinical research, but audit should always involve setting standards and evaluating whether they are met. Audit is likely to be most effective when routine and individualized, and acting on the results and re-auditing ('closing the audit loop') is an essential component. Promoting this therefore requires encouraging doctors to routinely measure relevant outcomes and preparing them to accept individualized feedback as constructive rather than critical (Haines & Donald 1998).

5. **Risk reduction** simply refers to minimizing the adverse effects of any service provided, i.e. ensuring that services are delivered as safely as possible. This might include regular patient surveys and critical incident reviews.

6. **Developing useful information systems**, i.e. to give clinicians and managers clinically relevant information to set and monitor standards and outcomes. This is probably the most fundamental but most difficult to implement aspect of clinical governance. Psychiatric case registers and other information systems rarely include clinically useful information on interventions and outcomes. If the latter were routinely measured and recorded, the information would be complementary to that from randomized and pragmatic clinical trials and would greatly aid clinical decision making. There are, however, three substantial hurdles to negotiate: monies are required to facilitate local development and national integration; gold standard outcomes are required to avoid simply compiling 'league tables' of hospital services; and security measures are necessary to preserve confidentiality.

Overall, clinical governance is closely linked to evidence-based medicine and critical appraisal. Unless adequately funded, however, it is likely to be as patchily and variably implemented as audit and community care have been until now.

EVIDENCE-BASED MEDICINE (EBM)

EBM can be defined as the 'conscientious, explicit and judicious use of the current best evidence in making decisions about the care of patients' (Sackett et al 2000). This includes formulating clinical questions in areas of uncertainty, reliably tracking down evidence, critically appraising the evidence in terms of scientific validity and clinical importance, implementing it (if valid and important), and monitoring this whole process. EBM is a simple concept with profound implications. It has been pioneered by clinicians interested in distinguishing useful clinical research from that which is invalid and/or unimportant, among an ever-increasing number of published articles that are potentially relevant to the practice of medicine. Evidence comes from both the medical literature and clinical experience, and can be usefully graded on a hierarchy. In considering treatments, for example, the most valid evidence – of efficacy – is likely to come from (in order): a meta-analysis of two or more randomized controlled trials (RCTs); an individual RCT; a controlled trial; an uncontrolled or 'open' trial; case series and case reports (Box 1.2). It is worth noting that clinical experience is an extended case series giving information on effectiveness rather than efficacy.

Box 1.2   A typical grading system for clinical research

Ia   evidence from a meta-analysis of RCTs
Ib   evidence from at least one RCT
IIa evidence from at least one controlled study without randomization
IIb evidence from at least one other well designed quasi-experimental study
III evidence from well designed non-experimental descriptive studies
IV   evidence from expert committee reports, opinions, clinical experience, etc.

CRITICAL APPRAISAL

Critical appraisal is arguably the most important component of EBM, as it concerns assessing the validity of the research and statistical techniques employed in studies and generating clinically useful information from them (i.e. separating the wheat from the chaff in the medical literature). This can be made relatively straightforward, with the use of the structured appraisal questionnaires for particular types of study developed by Sackett et al (2000) and others (see Chapter 4). There are also useful generic approaches (e.g. Fowkes & Fulton 1991).

Some components of research methodology are, however, more important than others, and all research has strengths and limitations, so that stating whether a particular piece of research is valid or not often requires some subtlety. This demands a working knowledge of research methods, the common sources of bias in each of the main approaches, and which statistical tests are appropriate in particular situations. In a sense, research methods and critical appraisal are mirror images of each other. One could use an in-depth knowledge of critical appraisal to design an acceptable study, and vice versa, but the two are best considered independently. Before one can even start critical appraisal, however, one needs to be able to identify information needs and ways of meeting them.

INFORMATION NEEDS IN CLINICAL PRACTICE

Contrary to how medical students are generally taught and how some doctors behave, uncertainty is almost universal in clinical medicine. Studies suggest that the average physician, when asked, could usefully seek clinically relevant information in two out of every three patients they see, and that such information would change their clinical decisions in one of every four cases (Covell et al 1985). We surveyed all the senior psychiatrists in southeast Scotland and most were able to identify three clinical questions to which they would like reliable answers. These were mainly about treatment, but included prognostic, diagnostic and aetiological issues (Lawrie et al 2000).

It takes practice to routinely identify areas of uncertainty and to ask clinical questions in a productive way. To be useful, in the sense of optimizing the chances of finding answers, such questions will be brief summaries of the clinical scenario and the information required, constructed in a way that makes searching for evidence likely to succeed. Specific questions will of course vary according to the situation, but productive questions tend to be composed of four parts ('the four-part clinical question'): the patient problem; the type of clinical issue or intervention being considered (e.g. diagnostic, prognostic or therapeutic); the comparison intervention (if appropriate); and the clinical outcome(s) of interest.

One way of encouraging colleagues to think in this way is to start a local evidence-based psychiatry journal club (EBPJC). This also develops critical appraisal skills, encourages the implementation of evidence-based clinical practice, and could facilitate clinical governance. Experience suggests that successful EBPJCs follow a fairly set pattern, as described by the Centre for Evidence-Based Mental Health (CEBMH, p. 9). Clinical questions are formulated at the beginning of each week's session. Suitable articles are then identified – searching should take no longer than a few minutes (with practice) and can be done there and then if a laptop computer with access to the main databases is available. If there is more than one suitable article then the most promising is selected by discussion with the group. Copies of the selected article will be made for EBPJC attenders the following week. About 45 minutes is spent appraising and discussing the paper each week. Once an EBPJC has been running for 2–3 weeks, this cycle should be self-perpetuating. Clinical questions about specific patients (e.g. those causing concern) are usually best, but it is always possible to appraise any journal article (cf. a traditional journal club). Regular attenders will quickly build up a file of reliable answers to commonly asked questions and authoritative sources for easy future reference.

INFORMATION SOLUTIONS

There are a number of approaches to trying to answer clinical questions reliably (e.g. Lawrie & Geddes 1998). The single most reliable resource for treatment questions is the Cochrane Library. This is the main output of the Cochrane Collaboration, named after Archie Cochrane and begun in 1992, which is an international endeavour to systematically find, appraise and review RCTs with the aim of conducting and maintaining up-to-date meta-analyses of RCTs in all forms of healthcare intervention. These meta-analyses are readily available to clinicians and other decision makers at all levels of healthcare systems through an electronic library, which is published quarterly and regularly updated and comprises:

1. The Cochrane Database of Systematic Reviews (CDSR)
2. The York Database of Abstracts of Reviews of Effectiveness (DARE)
3. The Cochrane Controlled Trials Register (CCTR)
4. The Cochrane Review Methodology Database (CRMD).

The Cochrane Library only considers treatment in any detail and is as yet rather patchy. The journal *Evidence-Based Mental Health* (EBMH) is probably the next best source of information, as it provides one-page summaries of recently published studies that meet quality criteria in all clinical areas, each quarter. This is a very useful secondary information source, but was only started in 1998 and does not place new papers in the context of all previously published papers. (An evidence-based medicine journal and the American College of Physicians Journal Club give some psychiatric coverage further back and are available on an annually updated compact disc called Best Evidence.)

Several computerized databases are available for literature searching. The most useful for those working in the mental health field are MEDLINE, the Bath Information Database Service (BIDS) and PsychLit. MEDLINE only covers the published literature from 1966, BIDS from 1980, and PsychLit from 1990. Considerable skill is required to reliably and quickly identify all potential articles of relevance in each database, as there is little quality control and each covers probably only about 40% of the literature on a particular topic. However, two new electronic sources of pre-evaluated papers from a wider range of publications have recently become available (see Resources, p. 9) and the CEBMH is actively establishing a database of 'critically appraised topics' and an electronic library for mental health (see Resources, p. 9).

It is unrealistic to expect individual clinicians to perform these searches for each and every question they may have. In addition, searches will commonly identify so many articles that it is difficult to decide which to use, or no relevant articles at all. There is therefore a need for reliable, regularly updated summaries of the best available evidence in a given clinical area. The *British Medical Journal* (BMJ) and the American College of Physicians (ACP) have recently collaborated to produce 'Clinical Evidence', which summarizes all the evidence for common treatment questions and will be updated every 6 months (see Resources, p. 9).

There remains a need for evidence-based guides to all aspects of the clinical management of common psychiatric disorders. The late 1990s was the age of clinical guidelines, which are 'systematically developed statements to assist practitioner and patient decisions about the appropriate healthcare for specific clinical circumstances'. They should involve various professionals and other 'stakeholders', be based on systematic reviews of all the available evidence, and explicitly grade recommendations according to the quality of the supporting evidence. Even reliable guidelines can, however, be difficult to implement. Explicit recommendations, dissemination with the active participation of 'stakeholders' and rigorous monitoring are the keys to success. If these approaches are taken guidelines can change medical practice for the better, particularly where a wide variety of treatment approaches is used (Woolf et al 1999). So far, psychiatric guidelines have rarely been systematic, but look out for papers and reports from the National Schizophrenia Guideline Group and NICE/SHTAC.

RESOURCES

Table 1.1 gives the Internet addresses of some of the resources we find most useful, together with some relevant background information.

Table 1.1 Useful Internet sources

Resource	Address	Information available
Bandolier	http://www.ebando.com	General information about evidence-based medicine
BioMedNet	http://www.biomednet.com	A search facility for pre-evaluated quality papers
Centre for Evidence-Based Mental Health	http://www.cebmh.com	General information on evidence-based medicine, with lots of useful links
Clinical evidence	http://www.evidence.org	The electronic version of the evidence summary produced by the BMJ/ACP
Cochrane Library	http://www.update-software.com	see text
Critical appraisal skills programme	http://www.phru.org/casp	Information about appraisal generally, as well as workshops etc.
US National guideline clearing house	http://www.guideline.gov	Evidence-based practice guidelines and evaluation
NHS centre for reviews and dissemination	http://www.york.ac.ukinst/crd	How to conduct systematic reviews, with examples
National Institute for Clinical Excellence (NICE)	http://www.nice.nhs.uk	Guidelines
Ottawa hospital library services	http://www.ogh.on.ca/library/ebm_e.htm	Comprehensive list of worldwide EBM resources
PubMed	http://www.ncbi.nlm.nih.gov/PubMed	Free access to MEDLINE with evaluation
Scottish Guidelines Development Programme	http://www.show.scot.nhs.uk/sign	Evidence-based clinical guidelines
User's Guide to the Literature	http://www.hiru.mcmaster	Guides to appraisal and tools to support it
Wisdom	http://www.shef.ac.uk/uni/projects/wrp1	Information on governance, appraisal and EBM

REFERENCES AND FURTHER READING

Cochrane A 1972 Effectiveness and efficiency: random reflections on health services. BMJ Books, Cambridge (Reprinted 1989)

Covell DG, Uman GC, Manning PR 1985 Information needs in office practice: are they being met? Annals of Internal Medicine 103: 596–599

Davis DA, Thomson MA, Oxman AD, Haynes RB 1995 Changing physician performance. A systematic review of the effect of continuing medical education strategies. Journal of the American Medical Association 274: 700–705

Fowkes FGR, Fulton PM 1991 Critical appraisal of published research: introductory guidelines. British Medical Journal 30: 1136–1140

Haines A, Donald A 1998 Making better use of research findings. British Medical Journal 317: 72–75

Lawrie SM, Geddes JR 1998 Evidence-based medicine and psychiatry. In: Johnstone EC, Freeman CPL, Zealley AK (eds) Companion to psychiatric studies. Harcourt Brace, Edinburgh

Lawrie SM, Scott AIF, Sharpe MC 2000 Evidence-based psychiatry: do psychiatrists want it and can they do it? Health Bulletin (Edinburgh) 58: 25–33

Sackett DL, Straus SE, Richardson WS, Rosenberg W, Haynes RB 2000 Evidence-based medicine: how to practise and teach EBM, 2nd edition. Churchill Livingstone, Edinburgh

Scally G, Donaldson LJ 1998 Clinical governance and the drive for quality improvement in the new NHS in England. British Medical Journal 317: 61–65

Woolf SH, Grol R, Hutchinson A, Eccles M, Grimshaw J 1999 Potential benefits, limitations and harm of clinical guidelines. British Medical Journal 318: 527–530

REVISION MCQs

Q1 Clinical governance includes the following:

(a) Clinical audit
(b) The development of clinical guidelines
(c) Continuing medical education
(d) Revalidation
(e) Evidence-based medicine

Q2 Evidence-based medicine:

(a) Is only concerned with medical treatments
(b) Includes asking clinical questions and monitoring one's performance
(c) Includes assessing the scientific validity and clinical importance of published research

(d) Recommends using only treatments based on evidence from controlled trials

(e) Disregards clinical experience

Q3 Critical appraisal:

(a) Is part of clinical governance
(b) Is a key component of the practice of evidence-based medicine
(c) Is the process of assessing the scientific validity of published research
(d) Can only be done by academics trained in research methods
(e) Requires an in-depth understanding of medical statistics

Q4 The Cochrane Collaboration:

(a) Is only concerned with treatment
(b) Produces an electronic library
(c) Includes only systematic reviews and meta-analyses
(d) Covers almost all currently used medical treatments
(e) Was established in 1992

Q5 The following statements are true of evidence-based information sources:

(a) A literature search is best preceded by the formulation of a four-part clinical question
(b) MEDLINE covers most of the published treatment studies in a given field
(c) Evidence-based journal clubs are run similarly to traditional journal clubs
(d) The EBMH journal puts new studies in the context of all previous studies
(e) Clinical guidelines are best derived from consensus meetings

ANSWERS

A1

(a) True
(b) True

(c) False (CPD not CME)
(d) False (not as yet)
(e) False (clinical effectiveness is related to EBM but not the same)

A2

(a) False (EBM equally applies to diagnosis, prognosis, etc.)
(b) True
(c) True
(d) False (EBM recommends using the best available evidence)
(e) False (although clinical experience is at the bottom of the evidence hierarchy)

A3

a) False
b) True
c) True
d) False (although research experience is helpful)
e) False (a knowledge of what sorts of test are appropriate in certain situations is enough)

A4

(a) True
(b) True
(c) False (Cochrane also registers trials in progress and high-quality reviews)
(d) False (only a fraction of all procedures are as yet considered)
(e) True

A5

(a) True
(b) False (only 30–40% of the relevant studies are covered)
(c) False
(d) False
(e) False

2

Research methods

Research is simply the systematic study of particular phenomena. Clinical research is an essential part of modern medicine. New treatments must be rigorously evaluated to protect patients (and to avoid wasting taxpayers' money). Health services research can optimize the delivery of medical care to patients. Even aetiological studies and basic laboratory research (of molecules, cells and animals) – sometimes called 'blue skies' research – have the overall aim of improving detection and treatment, with the ultimate goal of prevention. Many doctors, and perhaps psychiatrists in particular, do not seem to appreciate this and misunderstand the scientific process. It is true that progress is often painfully slow, but it is still progress and one can never know when the next major breakthrough will be made.

There are many good reasons why we need clinical research and at least some clinical researchers. There is also a rationale for expecting all doctors to know how to do research. A working knowledge of research methodology helps one to quickly understand the general thrust of a piece of research and to critically appraise the methods employed. This may help pass exams, but more importantly will allow clinicians to make up their own minds about the value of what they read in journals, books and drug company advertising for the rest of their career. There are even powerful reasons for all doctors getting research experience and continuing to do at least some. Designing and interpreting studies requires and fosters clear thinking. Actually doing some research is the best way of learning about it, and analysing the results is the best way of understanding statistics. Even being involved in a bad research project, which can lead to cynicism and resentment, may educate one in how not to do things. At the very least all doctors should be auditing the services they provide, in a bid to continually improve them.

This chapter will briefly consider how to go about doing research, describe the main clinical research methods in some detail, highlighting the main advantages and limitations of each, and close with a general description of the main considerations when interpreting the results of studies. Examples from the psychiatric literature will be used throughout.

DESIGNING A RESEARCH PROJECT

A curious and critical mind, careful planning and a determination to finish the study are necessary and sufficient for many research projects. A grant and assistance are not essential for clinical audit, surveys and case–control studies, although they do help. On the other hand, sizeable grants and research teams are generally required for cohort studies, clinical trials and technological investigations.

The first step is to **get an idea**. Ideas may arise from clinical observations, discussions with other staff, or reading the journals. Published articles often discuss what further studies are required. Simply attempting to replicate a particular study with minor alterations to clarify one issue can be an important contribution. Turning the idea into a question may help focus the idea by clarifying the aims and hypotheses, and suggest a research design. It can be helpful to think in terms of the four-part clinical question (see Chapter 1), i.e. patient problem, intervention, outcome and control subjects or interventions. Note that one idea or question is preferable, as it is more likely to be thoroughly addressed than if answers to two or more are attempted.

One must next **review the relevant literature**, preferably systematically, as truly original ideas are very rare. Reading previous papers can be a very time-consuming process, which irritates but is time well spent. It will identify what needs to be done, identify the strengths and weaknesses of particular research designs, what measures are potentially relevant, etc. If there is no recent good review article then you should write one.

Next, consider the advantages and disadvantages of the various research designs to answer your question, meet your aim or test your hypothesis. You must **realistically evaluate what you are able to do**. What sorts of patients and controls, and how many of them, do you have access to? It is wise to study the sorts of patients you are likely to see anyway in your clinical work. How much time will you have? If, for example, you have 2 hours a week for research, and each subject's measures will take an hour, it will take you at least a year to recruit and assess 50 patients and 50 controls. It is a good idea to construct a rough timetable for important stages of the research – ethical and grant applications, the pilot study, starting and completing data collection, data analysis and submission for publication – always allowing for the fact that it will take longer than you think owing to fatigue, holidays, subjects failing to turn up, etc. Will you have any help? One assistant will halve the time required, support you during the inevitable bad times, and will be able to ensure that any measures have 'inter-rater reliability' (see Chapter 3) if that is required.

You must now **write a research protocol** (Box 2.1). At this stage it is worth consulting an experienced researcher and/or statistician if you can and have not already done so. They will help to focus your idea, clarify the design and advise on sensible statistics. A protocol is essential for planning the study properly and will serve as a template for any ethical approval or grant applications you need to apply for.

A protocol starts with an **introduction**. This should discuss the issue you are addressing, briefly summarize the main findings and limitations of previous studies, and describe the aims of your study. If you are attempting to answer a particular question, as is preferable, you should predict what you expect to find and rephrase the prediction as a negative ('the null hypothesis'), e.g.

Box 2.1   A typical study protocol and hints on how to write it

1. Title	Keep it brief
2. Introduction	Why do the study?
	Previous and pilot studies
	Aims and/or hypotheses
3. Methods	Design (e.g. case–control)
	Subjects (who, where from and how defined)
	Inclusion and exclusion criteria
	Measures (demographics, disease descriptors, symptoms, exposures and outcomes)
	Statistical tests
	Power calculation
4. References	Essential references only
5. Patient information and consent forms	In lay language

there is no difference between cases and controls on ... This is because, strictly speaking, statistical comparisons are attempts to disprove the null hypothesis, rather than to prove something (see Chapter 3). In writing the introduction you may find it helpful to ask yourself, 'why does this study need to be done, at this time and in this way?'

The protocol should then describe the precise **methods** you intend to employ, particularly how you will identify and define **subjects**, the measurements you plan to make and the main statistical techniques you will use. Cases and controls should be as representative as possible of the entire populations from which they come. Inpatients are accessible and may be typical of admitted patients if they are a random sample of admissions or a consecutive series of admissions over a decent length of time, but are likely to have more severe and chronic illnesses than the average patient. A random sample of the entire caseload in a given locality is therefore generally preferable. Controls are usually even more difficult to identify and recruit. Hospital staff are often willing to help but are, by definition, employed, whereas many patients are not. Advertising for controls tends to attract people with a psychiatric history themselves or in their relatives. A random sample of the population is ideal but rarely practical. Often, the best compromise is to ask patients to identify friends and genetic or non-genetic relatives who may be able to participate, but a number of biases can be introduced in this way (see p.44). Ultimately, one has to decide which variables need to be controlled and how this can be most practically achieved. There is sometimes value in recruiting two or even more control groups, but this increases the workload and inevitably reduces statistical power.

The psychiatric diagnosis in cases must be verified in some way. This is often done by simply stating that patients meet certain diagnostic criteria for a particular disorder. This is easy, but easily biased. Case-note information varies in quality and comprehensiveness, patients can be 'squeezed' to fit certain categories, and comorbid conditions (which may need to be excluded) are easily missed. There are reliable ways of eliciting information from case-notes to generate **standardized diagnoses,** but actually interviewing all the subjects is preferable. A number of structured psychiatric interviews are available for this purpose – depending on whether you are interested in psychosis or 'neurosis' – but these can take an hour or more to complete. Some diagnostic schedules can also be used by trained lay interviewers, but this obviously requires time and money (see Duffy et al 1998 for further details).

Inclusion and exclusion criteria are usually based on diagnosis and demographics, such as age. Do not make inclusion criteria too restrictive or exclusions too numerous, as your study will lose representativeness and the ability to examine any differences within your patient group, and may well suffer from the 'disappearing patient' phenomenon. Inclusions are best kept to the diagnosis of interest, and exclusions limited to important conditions such as neurological disease. This will help to ensure that you have a large enough and representative sample. The effects of potentially confounding (see glossary) demographic variables and comorbid disorders (such as substance abuse) can then be examined directly. Indeed, identifying any within-group differences according to particular confounders may provide important supplementary information.

You must then describe the **measurements** you plan to make. Measures should ideally be reliable, valid, objective and standard. Only directly relevant data should be collected, to minimize the amount of time it takes you and the subjects to complete the study. Using at least some of the measures used in some of the previous studies will aid comparison and clarification. It is not possible to describe all the potential measuring scales (let alone technology-based observations) of interest in psychiatric research in a short chapter such as this (see Duffy et al 1998 for more details); some principles and some of the more commonly used scales are, however, worth a brief mention. Basic demographics (age, sex, social class) can be obtained from simply asking the subjects, although some descriptors (e.g. intelligence) will require specific scales. Relevant disease parameters, such as duration, medication and number of admissions, can be easily and fairly reliably obtained from case-notes. These variables may either confound any associations or modify the effects you discover, either in general or in particular subgroups of subjects (see Confounding, p. 48). Important potential exposures (or causative factors), confounders and outcomes all need to be measured, but the precise nature and number of each will depend on what you are studying.

Symptom severity is generally worth measuring and may be the outcome of primary interest. The most commonly used scales for psychotic symptoms are the Brief Psychiatric Rating Scale (BPRS) and the Positive And Negative Symptom Scale (PANSS). The

Hamilton Rating Scale for Depression (HRSD) and the Beck Depression Inventory (BDI) provide, respectively, objective and subjective measures of depressive symptoms. The Hospital Anxiety and Depression Scale (HADS) measures subjective depression and anxiety, and although it was developed for use in general hospitals it has found more widespread applications. Any of the various versions of the General Health Questionnaire (GHQ) are suitable for screening for psychiatric morbidity in the general population. The Krawiecka scale is a useful measure of the most frequent symptoms and signs in psychiatry. As doctors are generally showing an increasing interest in everyday functioning and quality of life, scales such as the Short Form 36 items (SF36) and the EuroQol and WHOQol are also worth considering.

If you are interested in something for which there is no scale or questionnaire, it is probably better to devise one yourself than to forcefully adapt something else. Devised instruments should be focused, brief and clear: for example, avoid confounding two issues in one question. If you need a simple measure of severity, for example, do not be afraid to ask subjects to mark a cross on a 10 cm line, as this is often surprisingly useful.

You will also need to give some thought to how the data will be recorded, stored, checked and analysed. This, and indeed all other aspects of your study, can and should be examined in a **pilot study**, which can determine whether your aims, recruitment and methods are realistic. Importantly, a pilot study will give you the best available information for a **power calculation** (see Chapter 3) to determine exactly how many subjects you will need. Briefly, a power calculation uses an estimate of the size of any effect or difference you expect to find to determine how many subjects will be needed to render such a result statistically significant (although you should note that any effect requiring relatively large numbers of subjects – say more than 30 in each group – is unlikely to prove to be *clinically* significant). Many grant-giving bodies and ethical committees now require evidence from pilot studies to ensure that ideas are feasible before giving monies or subjecting participants to projects that are unlikely to give clear-cut results. You should consider your main techniques of **statistical analysis**, which will depend on the types and likely distribution of your data (i.e. parametric or non-parametric statistics); whether you are simply describing subjects or comparing them (i.e. descriptive or inferential statistics); the number of groups; and any planned analysis of potential confounders (e.g. by subgroup, analyses of variance, regression) – see Chapter 3.

A comprehensive protocol will also contain a **patient information sheet and consent form**. Writing these will help you present your research idea in the sort of lay language that is required for ethical approval submissions (which always require information and consent sheets, and often place the greatest emphasis on them) and may be required for some grant-giving bodies.

The protocol will also provide you with the bulk of the introduction and methods sections of any papers you write to get your research published. The purpose of a paper is to communicate the essence of a research project so that it can be appraised in the context of others. An introduction should briefly summarize what is known and what needs to be in a particular area. A detailed methods section should be written so as allow your study to be replicated exactly (if anyone so desires). The results section should only give important positive and negative findings. The discussion should consider the results, strengths and limitations, and implications of your findings in the context of other studies. Thinking this far ahead at the planning stage may help to reduce avoidable biases and identify additional measures of potential confounders.

In summary, you should do something you are interested in, be realistic about what you can do, draft a protocol, get assistance, expect and rejoice in constructive criticism, do a pilot study, have a rough timetable, and stick at it. While you are waiting for the research to be published you could always try to answer the new questions it will inevitably give rise to.

THE ARCHITECTURE OF CLINICAL RESEARCH

There are essentially three types of clinical research:

1. **Descriptive observational studies**. Examples include case reports and series, audit projects, cross-sectional surveys of psychiatric morbidity and qualitative studies. As these are generally conducted without a control group for comparison, they are purely descriptive and are only suitable for hypothesis generation.

2. **Analytic observational studies**. Examples include case–control studies and (some) cohort studies. As these generally

compare two subject groups, i.e. cases and controls, they are suitable for hypothesis testing. Controls can be healthy subjects or those with a different disease. Ideally, the study and control groups are similar in all but the respect of main interest, e.g. similar in age and gender, but with and without a disease.

3. **Experimental studies**. The main examples in medicine are the controlled clinical trial and economic analyses, systematic reviews and meta-analyses of them. Something is given or done to the 'experimental' group but not to the controls, and any resulting differences in outcome are compared. As a result, causation can be inferred.

It can be seen that observational studies are precisely that – the study groups are only measured in various ways – whereas experimental studies involve actually doing something to one group. The distinction between descriptive and analytical studies is, however, far from absolute. Some clinical audits, surveys and qualitative studies include control groups, and some cohort studies do not. The necessity for and adequacy of a control group has to be evaluated on a study-by-study basis. Controls in audit studies tend to be the subjects themselves acting as 'historical controls', which can be seriously biased; controls in surveys are often recruited as a representative sample of the general population, which is ideal; and controls are simply not required in a cohort study of the outcome of a disease. In principle, any of these studies could be quantitative or qualitative, but the former is much more common in medicine and psychiatry.

CASE REPORTS AND CASE SERIES

These are simple descriptions of events in a single case or a number of cases. As a result they are very prone to all sorts of bias and chance associations. They are therefore usually only a means of identifying priorities or hypotheses for further and more comprehensive study. Psychoanalytical case studies, for example, are likely to contain much accurate and valuable insight but it is impossible to tell what is right from what is not. Put simply, a single case cannot prove anything ('one swallow does not make a summer') as coincidence is always possible. It is possible that a single case can disprove something – to paraphrase the philosophers David Hume and Karl Popper, seeing one black swan proves that all swans are not white – but this depends upon the measure being absolute rather than relative (is a grey swan black or white?).

Case reports and series should not, however, be dismissed (Farmer 1999), as they can be very influential (e.g. Freud's cases) and informative. For example, the associations between thalidomide and phocomelia, and *Helicobacter pylori* infection and peptic ulcer, were first described in single cases, as were a number of genetic anomalies. A description of the common features in a number of cases of a rare disease is likely to be the best available evidence on that problem. Open (uncontrolled) trials are case series that can obviate or demand further study. Further, every doctor's clinical experience is essentially an extended case series or, more accurately, a series of case series. It should be noted that case reports were by far the most common type of published medical research until comparatively recently, and that much of contemporary medicine is based on them and on clinical experience (Hennekens & Buring 1987).

CLINICAL AUDIT

Audit can be defined as the systematic and critical analysis of the quality of medical care. Strictly speaking, audit is not the same as research. Research attempts to establish what should be done in certain clinical situations, whereas audit measures what is actually happening – preferably against certain standards – attempts to improve usual practice, and then re-audits to close the 'audit loop/cycle'. The distinction can, however, be difficult to make, particularly as good clinical audit tends to employ many standard research methods.

Almost any aspect of clinical care can be audited. These can be usefully classified as audits of the *structure* of services (e.g. personnel, equipment), the *process* of care (e.g. note-keeping, investigations, treatments) and the *outcomes* of clinical interventions (e.g. morbidity and mortality). Audit studies of patient outcomes in everyday clinical practice are clearly important measures of local clinical effectiveness. Outcomes are arguably the most important measure, but can be difficult to define and measure. Such studies also require the recording of pertinent individual patient characteristics, to ensure that any outcome differences are not simply attributable to differences in 'case mix', i.e. that outcomes are related to treatments rather than to prognostic factors.

The essential components of audit are the development of a focus, agreeing on the standards to be achieved and the criteria for judging them, the collection of data, acting on the results and re-auditing (potentially ad infinitum). The particular methods employed will depend on the focus. Standards may be tailored to external recommendations or local desires. If they are identified and disseminated early, as is usually recommended, the initial audit is more likely to find desirable results but less likely to find subsequent improvements. If the effect of the audit is of prime interest, however, standards may be best developed after the first audit, so that the true effect of introducing them can be studied. One might aim first to improve the standard of psychiatric record-keeping, in which case hospital records will clearly have to be used. Generally, however, simply using case-notes is unsatisfactory, as doctors are notoriously unreliable in completing them, let alone comparably. A specific data-recording sheet is generally required and needs to be routinely completed for all patients. The data should ideally be objective ('hard'), to optimize reliable recording, but qualitative audits and subjective measures (e.g. patient satisfaction) are feasible and may be valuable.

Audit studies are generally uncontrolled. In a sense, if re-auditing is complete the first audit results could be regarded as a control for the second audit, but such 'historical controls' are very unreliable as so many other influences are brought to bear on services, patients and outcomes over time. Historical controls tend to overestimate the effects of new services. Audit is therefore best regarded as complementary to the results from RCTs and pragmatic clinical trials (Brugha & Lindsay 1996).

To date, psychiatric audits have concentrated on process issues such as emergency admission rates, the use of the Mental Health Act, prescribing habits (especially antipsychotic drug doses), adverse incidents and discharge procedures. The Royal College of Psychiatrists Research Unit has initiated national (UK) audits of the care programme approach and the management of violence. The vast majority of projects have concentrated on in-patients, but there is no reason not to expand these into outpatient and primary care settings. Equally, audits of structure (e.g. skill mix in the multidisciplinary team) and outcomes (e.g. deliberate self-harm, suicide) should be more common. One of the main problems to be overcome, for audit in psychiatric and all medical settings, is getting clinicians to appreciate the potential value (indeed necessity) of audit in constructively shaping rather than critically dictating clinical practice – as with clinical guidelines. Audit, like evidence-based medicine, has impressive face validity but a need to prove its worth.

SURVEYS

Surveys are generally cross-sectional studies of the prevalence and associations of a disorder. If they are conducted twice, incidence and predictors may be studied. Establishing the prevalence and incidence of a newly recognized or defined disorder does not require a control group and can usefully inform health service planning. Identifying the associations of a disorder can be achieved by comparing rates in different localities, or by comparing the associations in those with and without the disorder. Two-phase surveys generally screen a sample of the general population (e.g. with the General Health Questionnaire) and then conduct more detailed measures in the cases and a sample of controls from the population without the disorder. These associations can only generate hypotheses, however, as any exposure or risk factor is being determined after the onset of disorder and the temporal sequence is uncertain (the 'chicken and egg' problem). For example, psychiatric disorder is associated with poverty, but poverty may either follow or cause psychiatric disorder. The only exception to this rule is when exposures are unalterable over time, such as eye colour or blood group, or other factors present from birth.

There are various measures of disease frequency (see Chapter 3) but they are all measured in ratios, i.e. the numerator of interest is divided by the denominator of the whole population. (Rates are a special type of ratio that includes a time component.) It is, for example, meaningless to say that there are more patients with schizophrenia in England than in Scotland, as this compares numerators rather than ratios. This is sometimes called the **floating numerator fallacy**. The prevalence of a disease in a population can be determined by a cross-sectional survey at a particular point in time or over a period of time (the period prevalence). Establishing the incidence of a disease, however, requires two surveys, or some other follow-up technique, to establish the number of new cases that develop in a population over a certain length of time.

The key to conducting a good survey is ensuring that the population studied is representative of all the population, i.e. avoiding **sampling bias** and **response bias**. The best way to eliminate bias is to take a random sample (using random number tables) of the general population, but this is easier said than done. Census data rapidly become out of date as people move, the electoral roll does not include people who have not paid their 'community charge', and the telephone directory is still somewhat skewed towards the upper social classes. Although these problems do not invalidate these techniques, such limitations should be borne in mind. Psychiatric patients are probably overrepresented in all three categories, and of course are not available at all if they are in prison or hospital. A false association found through surveying an unrepresentative sample is known as **Berkson's fallacy**. For example, the observation that (hospitalized) patients with schizophrenia rarely had epilepsy led to the introduction of ECT, but was a fallacy (presumably because epileptics would be in general hospitals).

It is probably impossible to get a 100% response rate, but response can be maximized by attention to the methods of contacting subjects and the measures employed. Telephone or personal contact for a relatively brief interview may be more successful than simply sending questionnaires through the post. Intriguingly, response bias may differ between populations: as a rule psychiatric patients tend to be less likely to reply to a survey than controls, whereas medical patients are more likely to respond. For this reason, particularly in psychiatric surveys, more than one method of case ascertainment should be used to try to identify all the cases with a particular disorder in a given population (e.g. examine general practice and hospital records). This will also give valuable information on the characteristics of non-responders.

An **ecological study** is a special type of survey, also known as a correlational study, where whole populations rather than individuals are studied, often through the use of one or more computerized databases. The latter is known as record linkage. These are useful in generating hypotheses but cannot reliably identify any factor as a true cause, as other factors may account for an association. Incorrect conclusions about associations in ecological studies are called the **ecological fallacy**, as associations at a population level do not necessarily hold at an individual level. For example, regional suicide rates are *positively* correlated with numbers of consultant psychiatrists (as deprived areas have more of both).

QUALITATIVE STUDIES

Most medical research is quantitative, in the sense that the variables are 'objectively' measured in numerical terms. Qualitative studies, where measures are subjective (e.g. attitudes), are, however, seen as increasingly important. Qualitative research is concerned with personal meanings, experiences, feelings, values and other types of opinion. This is not necessarily 'soft' or 'unscientific'. The data are usually gathered with semistructured individual interviews, in focus group sessions and/or by simple observation. Objectivity can be ensured by taping these sessions and obtaining independent ratings by trained observers. It is worth noting that qualitative studies may complement and even inform quantitative approaches by, for example, helping in questionnaire development where relevant variables are not initially apparent.

Such an approach may be of particular value in psychiatry (Buston et al 1998). For example, psychiatrists' prescribing behaviour, the reasons for patients' non-compliance with treatment, and the stigmatization of psychiatric disorders are all complex issues that are likely to be differently determined in particular individuals or groups. Each of the main approaches to qualitative data collection has advantages and disadvantages. An individual interview elicits specific opinions but may not generalize to 'real life'. A focus group can examine group norms and the arguments for and against particular beliefs, but minority views may be obscured. Direct observation gives accurate information on ordinary events in natural settings, but without personal detail. The best methods to employ will depend on the phenomenon under investigation, but may well include more than one technique.

These techniques and opportunities have, however, been largely neglected in psychiatry, as in the rest of medicine. Examples are so few that it is worth running through the critical appraisal criteria (Sackett et al 2000) as pointers to research design. When evaluating a qualitative study, one should look for a clearly formulated question; an appropriate sampling of subjects and/or settings; a clear account of the researchers' perspective; a detailed account of data collection (preferably from more than one source

Table 2.1 Summary features of descriptive observational studies

Type of study	Essential features	Advantages	Disadvantages
Case report	Observations in a single case	Cheap and easy way of generating hypotheses	No comparison group, so cannot test hypotheses
Case series	Disease characteristics in a number of cases	May be best information on very rare diseases	No comparison group, so cannot test hypotheses
Audit	Examines service provision	Gives information on local effectiveness	Using historical controls is prone to bias
Survey	Measure rates of disease	Identify patterns of disease	Cannot distinguish cause and effect
Ecological study	Measure associations of disease	Can use pre-recorded data	Describe populations rather than individuals
Qualitative study	Elicits opinions	Can illuminate complex issues	Difficult to plan the data collection and analysis

and reliably rated) and how themes were derived from the data; credible results that address the original question; direct quotation; and the explicit consideration of alternative explanations.

The main limitations of qualitative research are that a researcher's interests are likely to influence what data are collected, and that it is difficult – if not impossible – to plan the data collection and analysis if one does not know what the characteristics of the data are likely to be. Proponents of the qualitative approach argue that these limitations are also common in quantitative research, to a much greater degree than most researchers like to acknowledge. The fact that analytical studies are generally designed to test specific hypotheses is their main advantage over descriptive studies. Table 2.1 summarizes the features of the various types of descriptive observational study.

CASE–CONTROL STUDIES

A case–control study is an observational analytic comparison of subjects with and without a particular disorder (Hennekens & Buring 1987). Cases with a disease and controls without it are compared on the rates of *previous* exposure to a measure of interest. These are now the most common types of study in medicine, as they can be relatively easy but often deliver important results. Many exposures can be investigated simultaneously and rare diseases can be examined. They are, however, prone to many types of bias and confounding, as information on the exposure(s) is obtained *retrospectively*.

Researchers must usually therefore rely on subjects' memories, or the accuracy and completeness of medical records. Memory can be unreliable, particularly where affected individuals or their relatives are more likely to remember potential causes of their illness ('search after meaning'), resulting in **recall bias**. The general difficulty in assessing exposures retrospectively is often called **information bias**. For example, mothers with schizophrenic children may be more likely to remember obstetric complications than those whose children are unaffected (recall bias), and obstetric notes are more likely to record some events than others (information bias).

The selection of cases and controls is particularly important. They should be representative of the general population of cases and controls, and ideally differ only in terms of the disease of interest. 'Matching' for important possible confounders, such as age and sex etc., has obvious value and reduces the number of subjects required. It is, however, very difficult to achieve close matching without seriously limiting the numbers of suitable subjects, and it is impossible to examine the effects of any matched variables in the statistical analysis. Matching should therefore only be attempted if the effect of a confounder is very large and cannot be quantified (see Confounding, p. 48).

Subjects should also be selected independently of the exposure(s) of interest. This is best achieved by randomly selecting samples from all the cases and potential controls in a given location, e.g. through true random sampling; from the second stage of a survey; or by 'nesting' a case–control study within a cohort study. Otherwise, **selection bias** is likely to falsely increase any difference in exposure frequencies. For example, patients with depression admitted to a psychiatric hospital are likely to differ from all patients with depression on the well-known variables that influence detection and referral in general practice. Selecting cases in contact with medical services is, however, the most common method as it is the most practical, but it behoves researchers to carefully consider potential sources of bias (Lewis & Pelosi 1990). Controls can be recruited as patients with another disorder, from the general population, or as relatives or friends of the cases. Each approach has advantages and disadvantages: other patients are accessible but ill; the general public are healthy but less likely to take part; and personal contacts of the cases are likely to be of similar background, and may be so similar as to reduce the association of interest – although they can also be selected by cases as they are 'super-healthy', thereby increasing any differences.

Selecting cases in contact with medical services also makes it difficult to determine whether any given exposure is associated with severity or chronicity, rather than the disease per se. Indeed, this is a common limitation of case–control studies. Unless the effects of an exposure on such features of the disorder are known, one cannot determine whether any characteristic is related to the cause or the prognosis of any illness. For example, obstetric complications may be related to an early onset of schizophrenia (and other neuropsychiatric disorders), rather than the disease itself. Similarly, as the exposure is assessed in retrospect it is often difficult to be sure whether any event occurred before or after the onset of disease. It is for this reason that researchers interested in the relationship between life events and depression place the greatest emphasis on independent events such as bereavement, rather than potentially related events such as becoming unemployed. Such an approach is, however, not always possible. Prospective case–control studies, in which newly diagnosed cases are identified in a specific time period, are an alternative but can be so time-consuming as to lose one of the main advantages of the case–control study. Temporal associations, and indeed the role of exposures in general, are usually best evaluated in cohort studies.

COHORT STUDIES

In a typical analytic cohort study subjects are classified by whether or not they have been exposed to a suspected risk factor for a disease, and then followed up for a period of time to determine the development of disease in each group. Prospective follow-up needs to be sufficiently long term (usually several years) and complete that enough subjects develop the disease of interest to allow meaningful comparisons of disease rates between the exposed and unexposed. Cohort studies can thus establish aetiology (causation). They can also be used to study multiple possible outcomes from a single exposure. As they generally require large samples, and are obviously time-consuming, cohort studies are best suited to studying relatively common diseases. Relatively rare disorders can, however, be suitable for cohort studies if subjects are at enhanced risk for other reasons (e.g. those with a strong family history of schizophrenia), or if an outcome is common among those exposed, i.e. if the 'attributable risk percent' (see Chapter 3) is high. Alternatively, retrospective cohort studies – where the cohort has already been exposed and developed the disease or not – can be conducted. These are particularly useful if the latent period between any exposure and the disease is long, where researchers would be likely to lose contact with large numbers of subjects. For example, a number of studies of neurodevelopment in schizophrenia have used data collected from national surveys of child development and linked them to registers of hospital admissions for schizophrenia. Such studies are relatively cheap and quick but depend upon data collected for other purposes, which may be incomplete and particularly deficient in information on potential confounders.

Readers should also appreciate that uncontrolled cohort studies can be usefully employed to generate valuable descriptive information, particularly on the prognosis of certain disorders and any adverse events (harm) associated with a particular intervention. Again, the cohort must be sufficiently large and followed for long enough for a number to develop the outcome of interest, which should be measured in all subjects. In addition, such cohorts should consist of representative samples of patients with a particular disorder and be gathered at a similar stage of the illness, preferably at onset.

The key distinction between cohort and case–control studies is that in (prospective) cohort studies the population is selected before the onset of disease or outcome of interest, whereas case–control studies generally occur afterwards. Cohort studies can therefore measure the exposure without any bias in relation to the disease. Clearly, however, the assignment of the disease/ outcome status could be biased unless follow-up is near complete and such data are rigorously defined ('hard'), or outcome assessors are blind to exposure status. Subjects who drop out of the study or move away and become uncontactable are likely to differ from those that do not (often because they have developed the disease of interest). Psychiatric diagnoses and outcomes are relatively 'soft' data and therefore need to be reliably, and preferably blindly, assessed. For example, deciding whether a particular subject has a

Table 2.2 Summary features of analytic observational studies

Type of study	Essential features	Advantages	Disadvantages
Case control	Subjects with and without a disease are compared on rates of exposure	Relatively few subjects required Suitable for rare diseases Can evaluate distant and multiple exposures	Prone to bias Inefficient for rare exposures Temporal relationships can be difficult to establish
Cohort	Exposed and non-exposed subjects are compared on rates of disease	Can evaluate rare exposures, temporal relationships and multiple outcomes Reduce bias	Expensive and lengthy Loss to follow-up threatens validity

psychiatric disorder or not should be based upon reliably elicited information from a structured psychiatric interview or case-note assessment. Retrospective cohort studies, in which exposure and disease status are measured by the researchers, have all the potential biases of a case–control study. Retrospective studies of prerecorded data have the advantage that the data are unlikely to be biased, but this information can always be biased in how it is obtained, e.g. tracing children who subsequently became psychiatric cases will only identify those in contact with psychiatric services, and especially those with recurrent admissions.

Finally, it is worth noting that case–control studies can sometimes be inserted into cohort studies, in a similar way to the second stage of a two-stage survey. Such 'nested' designs can reduce the costs of potentially expensive assessments. For example, blood samples from all subjects could be stored, but only analysed in the cases and a sample of non-cases at later date. Table 2.2 highlights the key features of case–control and cohort studies.

CLINICAL TRIALS

Clinical trials, also sometimes known as experimental or intervention studies, are used to evaluate the effects of a new treatment or a novel way of providing a service. They can be thought of as cohort studies, as subjects are identified by exposure status and followed to determine the outcome, although the exposure (intervention) is assigned by the researchers. Although some authorities appear to regard the clinical trial as synonymous with the 'gold standard' of the randomized controlled trial (RCT), there are in fact several types of clinical trial, just as there are various measures of therapeutic benefit.

The simplest clinical trial is 'open' or uncontrolled. These have their place, particularly in the early stages of drug development, but habitually overestimate the beneficial effects of an experimental treatment by an average of 20% (see Schulz et al 1995). For example, several open trials suggested that dialysis was useful in schizophrenia until an RCT showed it was not. The next, and generally the minimum acceptable, level of sophistication is the controlled trial, in which the 'controls' are given a placebo or standard treatment and a second (experimental) group is given the new treatment. However, controlled trials, without concealed randomization (see below), typically overestimate the benefits of new treatments by 40% (Schulz et al 1995).

There are even several types of randomized controlled trial (RCT). RCTs generally measure the effects of a treatment in groups of individual patients, but sometimes (particularly in evaluating service delivery or trials of prevention) the group is the unit of randomization. These are therefore sometimes called 'cluster trials'. These two types of RCT allow doctors to establish whether a treatment works in general ('efficacy'), but do not establish whether it works in everyday clinical practice ('effectiveness'). Trials of the latter include 'pragmatic trials' – RCTs in which all the individuals in a locality are included – and 'n-of-1 treatments trials', where a single patient receives two or more treatments sequentially.

It is the process and concealment of **randomization** that gives the RCT its status as the medical equivalent of a scientific experiment. The aim of randomization is twofold. First, assigning patients at random to one group or another should provide two more or less identical groups, in terms of both known and unknown possible confounders, so that any differences observed at the end of the trial can be ascribed to the different treatments. Secondly, the randomization order (if concealed) means that the investigators cannot filter particular patients into certain treatment groups. Otherwise, it is all too easy for doctors to pervert the randomization process, for example by recruiting patients with a relatively good prognosis to the new treatment arm, for the very best (keen to help) or worst (fraudulence) of reasons. The concealment of randomization should be maintained for the duration of the trial, so that the two groups are treated as equally as possible (apart from the intervention being examined). Ideally, an independent person (such as a statistician) should consult random number tables (or even toss a coin) to decide which treatment consecutive recruits will receive (see Pocock 1983 for further details). The results should be written on cards, which are sealed in opaque envelopes and only opened (preferably by an independent investigator such as the pharmacist) as each suitable patient is recruited. Both the randomization and the concealment of its result are crucial: without concealment the trial is not truly randomized.

The next important consideration in a trial is the treatment itself. If two drugs are being compared, doses may be fixed or flexible. Fixed doses are much more likely to generate truly comparable results, but inevitably mean that some patients will receive inadequate and others excessive doses. For example, haloperidol – the most common standard comparator drug in antipsychotic trials – is known to have an 'inverted U' efficacy curve (i.e. low and high doses have suboptimal benefits). Flexible dosing is more akin to clinical practice, which tailors individual patients' doses, but is often difficult to achieve without the investigators knowing what drug a particular patient is taking. In either case it is important to measure treatment compliance, either biochemically or by 'pill counting', as non-compliance can bias the results. In a comparison of talking treatments it is crucial that the time spent with a therapist is balanced in both groups, to control for non-specific therapeutic ('placebo') effects, and that the treatment is given in a structured and therefore repeatable fashion. Placebo effects can occur with any treatment given or taken with enough enthusiasm.

Ensuring that patients and doctors do not know which treatment is being given – **blinding** – reduces the potential biases of a patient's placebo response (in single blinding) and the doctor's sometimes overzealous desire to find a good new treatment (in double blinding). Even if drugs are presented similarly, however, patients and doctors can be 'unblinded' by side-effects, especially if these are distinctive. It is often useful, therefore, to ask patients and doctors to guess what treatments were being given to assess the success of the blinding. Better still, in 'triple blinding' the analysis of outcomes is conducted by independent researchers. This is clearly essential in psychotherapy trials, as it is difficult for patients to participate in therapy without knowing it (although they may not know what sort of therapy they are getting) and impossible for therapists to deliver a therapy without knowing what they are supposed to be doing. Non-blind outcome assessment is very prone to **observer bias**, which is the main threat to the validity of a clinical trial. If blinding is simply not possible for some reason, one should rely upon objective outcome measures that are less susceptible to observer bias.

The main outcomes of interest should be specified before the trial starts. It can often be difficult to identify outcomes that are statistically sensitive to change, clinically relevant, and also reflect everyday matters of importance to the patient. Dichotomous outcomes (e.g. dead/alive, employed/not) are easy to measure and of obvious significance. Moreover, they considerably simplify the required **intention-to-treat analysis**. Such an analysis considers the outcomes in every patient who was originally randomized to one or other treatment – in effect, trial dropouts are regarded as treatment failures, rather than ignored. A supplementary analysis of those who actually completed treatment can be added, but will overestimate the benefit of treatment. However, various scales may also be necessary to measure symptom changes, quantify any improvement in functioning, or measure quality of life. If so, any missing data from trial dropouts can be given the last known value ('last observation carried forward') or the mean for the group to permit an intention analysis, but these approaches are less reliable. Other considerations at the analysis stage include controlling for any (chance) uneven distribution of confounders between the groups, and subgroup analyses for potentially important prognostic indicators. However, a statistically significant difference in confounders may not be clinically relevant (and vice versa), and subgroup analyses should be prespecified to avoid chance findings from multiple hypothesis testing or 'data dredging'.

Cluster trials are a special type of RCT in which interventions are directed at groups rather than individuals. For example, if one wanted to establish the impact of an educational package on general practitioners' ability to detect and treat depression, randomizing patients would cause difficulty with blinding and other biases. It would be better to randomize GPs, or even whole practices, even though information could still leak out (e.g. on the golf course). The main problem with cluster randomization is that the data should be analysed in clusters (as the unit of randomization) rather than as individuals, and that a lot of clusters are needed to give sufficient statistical power to detect an effect of the new intervention if there is one.

Common problems with RCTs include failures of true randomization or concealment of the allocation (or failing to report them); a lack of blind treatment and/or outcome assessment; ignoring missing data; and using inappropriate or too many outcome measurements. Most trials in psychiatry tend to be small. Although it can be argued that any effects that only emerge in trials with more than 30 patients in each group are unlikely to be clinically important (Pocock 1983), randomization in small trials is unlikely to balance confounders and can therefore give rise to false-positive results. The rise of the multicentre 'mega-trial' in medicine is, however, a mixed blessing. On the one hand they give very accurate measures of the effects of treatments and confounders, which can at least be generalized to patients in all participating centres, but they may find statistically significant effects that are not clinically important.

The most common current criticism of RCTs, regardless of their methodological sophistication, is that subjects are highly selected and therefore unrepresentative of typical patient populations. In other words, they have good internal but poor external validity. The sort of patient who can give informed consent and is willing to participate in a study is quite likely to be different from the average patient, e.g. they tend to have a better prognosis. This is particularly true in psychiatry, where detained patients cannot ethically be included in trials. Patients in trials also usually have only one diagnosis, whereas comorbidity is common in medicine and many psychiatric patients also abuse alcohol and/or illegal drugs. It is therefore now standard practice to describe all the subjects considered for a trial and all those approached to participate, to allow one to determine whether exclusions or non-participation seriously threaten the generalizability of the results. An awareness of these issues has led to the rise of the 'pragmatic trial'.

Pragmatic trials include all patients with a particular disorder in a given location, and therefore have generalizability. The key component is that the treatment, patients and services are representative of what is or could reasonably be routinely available (Hotopf et al 1999). Otherwise, the pragmatic trial does not differ from the traditional type of RCT, although its scientific quality can be compromised. In particular, blinding may present problems and dropouts may be substantial. It should also be noted that if a new service is being evaluated in a pragmatic (or cluster) trial, enthusiastic and often highly trained professionals are generally employed to provide the treatment. This obviously favours the new service and does not allow for 'staff burnout', and so, strictly speaking, the health workers should also be randomized to the old or the new service.

An alternative approach to establishing effectiveness are so-called **n-of-1 trials**. In such a single case experiment two or more treatments are blindly given in succession to an individual patient (Guyatt et al 1986), who therefore acts as their own control. As long as the target of treatment is prespecified this can establish the best treatment for a particular individual, but not for anyone else. This approach, however, has the limitation of using a historical control and all the disadvantages of the crossover trial, of which the *n*-of-1 trial is a special example. **Crossover trials**, in which patients receive different interventions in turn, are now rarely used (unless the patients are very rare) as order effects and carryover (or hangover) effects are potential explanations for any apparent benefit and are difficult to exclude. Order effects are a common problem in many types of research, in that any differences between subjects on two or more occasions may be attributable to the order in which they received or did something, rather than the interventions themselves. Carryover effects refer to the specific problem in crossover trials, where a treatment may have long-lasting effects that obscure the effects of a subsequent treatment. Any 'washout' period between treatments needs to be long enough to separate the treatment effects, and the length of the treatment itself must be sufficient for it to work but not so long that natural remission is likely.

Table 2.3 summarizes the features of the different types of clinical trial.

ECONOMIC ANALYSES

Health economics can be applied to many aspects of healthcare but are most commonly applied to treatment. This helps to make decisions about the best use of resources by comparing the effects or 'outputs' of competing interventions in relation to their costs or 'inputs'. These then are examinations of efficiency, but are best considered with reference to studies of efficacy and effectiveness.

Table 2.3 Summary of the features of clinical trials

Type of study	Essential features	Advantages	Disadvantages
Open trials	All subjects are given one treatment	Cheap and easy	No controls
Controlled trials	Two treatments are compared	Relatively straightforward	No randomization
RCT	Randomization Blinding Intention-to-treat analysis	Randomization minimizes bias and confounding	Expensive, difficult and time-consuming May not generalize to clinical practice
Cluster trials	Groups of individuals are randomized	Can establish the efficacy of various health services	Often difficult to find enough groups to give power
Pragmatic trial	All patients in a location are randomized	Representative and generalizable test of effectiveness	Difficult to control, blind and avoid excessive dropouts
Crossover trial	Subjects are their own controls	Can study treatment of rare disorders	Historical controls Order effects Carryover effects
n-of-1 trial	A single subject	Can establish effectiveness in a particular case	As above

An economic analysis can be applied to audit, but is most reliably conducted alongside a randomized clinical trial.

The four main types of economic analysis are:

1. Cost minimization – in which only the inputs are considered, i.e. the costs of the treatment, as the outputs are assumed to be equal, e.g. using the cheapest of two equally effective treatments. This is related to the concept of 'technical efficiency', in that improvements are maximized for a given input.

2. Cost–benefit – in which all the inputs and outputs are simply measured in monetary terms, e.g. the costs of drugs, staff and services versus the costs of time off work with and without treatment. As clinical outputs are difficult to measure financially, one can ask patients how much they would be 'willing to pay' for the benefits from certain procedures, or to choose between pairs of interventions (in a 'conjoint analysis').

3. Cost-effectiveness – in which costs are related to a clinical output measure, such as life years gained, or another generic outcome measure. This allows comparisons of 'relative

(productive) efficiency' – maximizing a health outcome for a given cost per outcome – but cannot compare different outcomes or even choose between interventions providing more benefit at greater cost or less benefit at lower cost.

4. Cost–utility – in which an output, such as the quality of life adjusted year, combines quantitative and qualitative information of the amount of life gained and the relative quality of that to individuals. This is an interval measure, in that a score of, say, 10 is twice as good as one of 5. The use of such a common measure allows one to compare diverse interventions and choose between them, i.e. both 'productive' and 'allocative' efficiency are measured. This societal perspective also explicitly acknowledges 'opportunity cost', i.e. that spending on one intervention means that another cannot be implemented. The problem with this approach is that assigning values to different health states is very subjective, e.g. having a severe dementia may or may not be considered worse than death.

The information on inputs and outputs may not always be available from RCTs. Where this is the case economists model the probability of events (in a 'decision tree analysis') based on the best available data or expert opinion (Kernick 1998).

Designing or evaluating an economic analysis therefore requires consideration of both the underlying research approach and whether all relevant inputs – direct (medical) and indirect (societal) costs – and outputs are included. This is, however, dependent on various assumptions about the inputs to be included, the value at which they should be costed, and how they should be 'discounted' to allow for inflation, all of which may vary among different patient populations. The assumptions about these matters in any evaluation must therefore be explicit, and the results should be examined with a variety of alternatives in a 'sensitivity analysis'. A sensitivity analysis involves systematically examining the influence of uncertainties in these assumptions and variables. 'One-way analysis' examines plausible changes in one variable at a time (probably underestimating uncertainty), whereas 'extreme scenario analysis' sets variables to minimal and maximal values (probably overestimating uncertainty). The most realistic 'probabilistic analysis' involves simultaneously examining the effects of changing variables across plausible ranges in a number of 'Monte Carlo simulations'. For example, manufacturers of new antidepressants and antipsychotics often present evidence that these drugs are more cost-effective, despite higher cost, as the output of reduced side-effects or toxicity results in fewer and/or briefer hospital inpatient stays. However, not only are these rarely presented with sensitivity analyses, it is also unclear how these apparent cost-efficiency savings can be realized without closing hospital beds; but this is a complex and evolving area, as is health economics generally. The critical appraisal section of this book gives a detailed evaluation of an economics paper (with references for further reading), and readers are referred to Kernick (1998) and the recent series of 'economics notes' in the *British Medical Journal* of 1999 2000 for further details.

SYSTEMATIC REVIEWS AND META-ANALYSES

Systematic reviews and meta-analyses are syntheses of the available evidence in a particular research area. A systematic review gathers and cites all this evidence in a prespecified way; a meta-analysis generates a quantitative summary of the evidence. They are clearly complementary. Although a systematic review can have value without an accompanying meta-analysis, the reverse is less true. The two are increasingly important in all areas of medical research, for two main reasons. Any single study, even if rigorously conducted and analysed, is only an estimate of the true effect and needs to be independently replicated, but subsequent studies may not agree with the original for various reasons. Doctors can only be expected to keep up to date with a fraction of the millions of medical papers published each year, and therefore need access to high-quality review articles.

Traditional 'narrative' reviews, in journals or books, are often based on a selective citation or reading of the literature, and may also be out of date. A review is a study of studies (cf. a retrospective study) and, if it is based on only a selection of papers, is likely to be biased (analogous to selection bias). For example, the implementation of thrombolysis for acute myocardial infarction was delayed by about 10 years after a systematic review would have concluded it was beneficial, because the consensus was that thrombolysis was of little benefit. It has also been shown that doctors with links to the tobacco and drug industry tend to express relatively benign views about passive smoking and the risks of new drugs, respectively. It is likely that psychiatrists with close links to the drug industry have more positive views of the new antipsychotics and antidepressants than those who do not. Perhaps most concerningly, self-professed expertise is highly and negatively correlated with adherence to systematic reviewing principles, i.e. 'experts' are more likely to write biased reviews (Sackett et al 2000).

It is therefore difficult to overstate the importance of systematic reviews. They are becoming increasingly common and are an essential preliminary to research studies. Systematic reviews require:

1. The formulation of a specific question
2. Prespecification of the types of article to be included and excluded
3. Prespecification of important outcomes and any statistical analysis
4. Use of several search strategies to identify potentially relevant articles, e.g. from a number of computerized databases (as each only contains a minority of the papers in a given area), hand-searching of relevant journals, examining the references for other studies, and contacting researchers (and possibly drug companies) for other published and unpublished studies they know of
5. Identification of relevant articles and what data should be used (ideally cross-checked with at least one other reviewer to check reliability)
6. Citation of all the identified articles
7. A system for measuring the quality of individual studies.

Systematic reviews are not therefore to be entered into lightly. Trying to identify and locate all the relevant articles in a research area can be very time-consuming, and a particular concern is that missed studies may differ from those found. A common reason for this is the presence of publication bias. **Publication bias** is simply the phenomenon that studies with positive results are more likely to be published, as researchers are more likely to write up and submit articles with a positive result and (especially leading) journals are more likely to publish them (Egger & Davey Smith 1998). This is less of a problem with interventional studies than it used to be, as the leading journals have actively promoted the reporting of negative trials, and registering of clinical trials is increasingly prevalent, but remains a particularly important issue for reviewers of observational research. Publication bias can be evaluated with funnel plots or Galbraith plots (see Chapter 3), minimized by contacting other researchers in the field, and controlled in a meta-analysis by estimating the 'failsafe *n*' of negative 'desk-drawer' studies that would cancel any significant result.

It should, however, be noted that some narrative reviews still have a role to play – it is just that they should be regarded as opinion rather than fact. Broad reviews and editorials can put evidence in context, summarize large related fields of study (e.g. including harm, quality of life and the patients' perspective), and stimulate new thought.

Meta-analysis is complementary to systematic reviewing, as it combines studies mathematically to provide a summary 'best estimate' of any true effect. Individual studies may find different results for several reasons, e.g. measurement error, bias, confounding, inadequate power, etc. Simple 'vote-counting' summary techniques (e.g. nine studies find a difference, versus six which do not) do not include an assessment of study size or quality and have low power. Large studies, which are generally of higher quality and provide more precise estimates of any effect than do smaller studies (Schulz et al 1995), should have relatively more influence on a summary effect. This is achieved by 'weighting' studies according to size and/or quality (see Chapter 3). Thus, meta-analyses derive a quantitative summary of the effect size from two or more studies by statistically combining effect sizes weighted by study size/quality.

Note, however, that meta-analyses are far from infallible. They are unreliable if they are based on non-systematic literature reviews, because they are sensitive to publication bias, 'location biases' and 'inclusion bias'. Location biases increase or decrease the chances that certain articles will be found, according to the language used, the database, citation habits, any multiple publication and the data actually provided. Inclusion bias is the habit of reviewers of including data they agree with, and vice versa.

Meta-analyses are also unreliable if the event rates are low and the number of studies is small, and are obviously influenced by the quality of the original trials. These problems can result in 'heterogeneity', where the results from different groups of studies differ to a statistically significant extent, and the summary estimate is therefore unreliable. This may also arise if treatment effects vary according to particular patient characteristics, clinical settings, and even the year of the study, all of which are quite common. There are, as yet, no ways of combining the results of randomized and non-randomized clinical trials.

Meta-analysis was devised, and continues to evolve, to deal with the results from RCTs. They can be used to summarize effects from observational research but may give 'spurious precision' and may best be used to examine the various influences of distinct methodological factors in such instances. Particular care is needed in interpreting a meta-analysis that disagrees with the results from the largest RCT and when two or more meta-analyses of the same topic fundamentally disagree. None the less, the advantages of meta-analysis generally outweigh the problems. Some enthusiasts even think that all RCTs should give an updated (cumulative) meta-analysis in the discussion part of all papers.

Table 2.4 summarizes the main types of research study used in medicine.

INTERPRETING THE RESULTS OF STUDIES

Any research finding could, in theory at least, be true or false. False positives are sometimes called type I errors, and false negatives type II. A false finding can be attributable to chance (random error), 'reverse causality', bias or confounding. Observational studies are particularly prone to these problems, if the exposure is measured after the onset of disease. Prospective cohort studies and controlled clinical trials – which measure the exposure (or treatment) before the disease (or outcome) – are designed with these potential problems in mind, but may still suffer from them. Establishing such a temporal sequence is an important 'criterion of causality', as devised by Bradford Hill. The other criteria are a strong association (e.g. the odds of an aetiological association should be elevated threefold before a novel finding is taken seriously); a 'dose–response' relationship (i.e. those with a greater number of or more severe exposures are more likely to get the outcome); consistency with existing knowledge; and biological plausibility. These can be very helpful guides to whether an association is real or artefactual.

The role of **chance** is a general problem, dealt with largely by statistical techniques. It is, however, important to realize that stating a finding to be 'statistically significant' (usually as $P<0.05$) only means that such an association or difference would arise by chance less than 5% of the time (or once in every 20 times). This arbitrary significance level means that this is *unlikely* to have occurred by chance: it does not mean it did not. Power is an

Table 2.4 Summary of the features of the main types of medical research study

Type of study	Question addressed	Advantages	Disadvantages
Experimental		*Reliable answers*	*Expensive*
Meta-analysis and/or systematic review of RCTs	Treatment	Best available evidence of efficacy	Literature search must be exhaustive
Randomized controlled trials (RCTs)	Treatment	Reliable measure of efficacy, controlling for confounders	Does not measure effectiveness; may be ethical objections
Economic analysis (of RCTs)	Costs and/or utilities of interventions	Can help prioritize services	Dependent upon many assumptions
Pragmatic clinical trials	Treatment	Representative of all types of patient	Less reliable results than RCTs
Observational		*Relatively easy*	*Susceptible to bias*
Cohort study	Aetiology Harm Prognosis	Suitable for rare exposures and multiple outcomes	Unsuitable for rare diseases; follow-up must be complete
Case–control	Diagnosis Aetiology	Quick, inexpensive; suitable for rare diseases, distant and multiple exposures	Prone to bias and confounding; unsuitable for rare exposures
Clinical audit	All, but especially treatment	The best measure of your own population	Routine monitoring is resource intensive
Qualitative	Personal thoughts and feelings	Can study complex issues	Subjectivity is difficult to compare
Surveys	Disease frequency and associations	Helps plan services and generate hypotheses	Susceptible to bias and confounding; cannot evaluate timing of exposure
Case reports and series	Any (potentially)	Very simple	Prone to chance association

important issue here. If a study did not have enough power to detect a finding but does so, technically it is a chance result. If a study did not have enough power to find a result and did not find it (usually because the sample was too small and the random error correspondingly large), type II error is possible. A particular problem arises if several statistical tests are done on a data set, as a statistically significant finding ($P<0.05$) will be generated for every 20 tests by chance alone. This can happen if research questions, hypotheses and statistical analyses are not carefully planned, leading to multiple hypothesis testing. In frankly bad research, researchers may simply 'dredge' or 'torture' their data set until a result is found. These issues are considered in greater detail in Chapter 3.

Reverse causality is a particular problem for descriptive and case–control studies. This simply means that an association between an exposure and a disease arises because the disease causes the exposure, rather than vice versa. For example, the original observation from an ecological study that patients with schizophrenia tended to be of lower social class was latterly shown to be because schizophrenia causes poverty. Similarly, life events (such as divorce) could be a cause or an effect of depression, possibilities which are very difficult to distinguish unless one conducts a cohort study or focuses on truly 'independent life events', such as bereavement.

Bias and confounding are more complex issues that require more detailed consideration. It can be difficult distinguishing the two, but it may be helpful to think of bias as something that is introduced by poor research technique, and to regard confounding as a relationship in nature that must be controlled for in good research designs.

Bias

Bias can be defined as 'any process at any stage of inference which tends to produce results or conclusions that differ (systematically) from the truth' (Sackett 1979). There are several types of bias that can arise at any stage of research (Sackett mentions 35), but the most important are selection (recruitment) and observation (measurement) biases. These can be usefully considered according to whether they are introduced (primarily) by researchers or by subjects themselves (Table 2.5).

Selection bias
Selection (or recruitment) bias arises through the identification and/or recruitment of an unrepresentative study population. This is particularly important in observational studies, especially in descriptive research, but potentially important in any study, e.g.

Table 2.5   The main types of bias in medical research

Selection bias	
Sampling	Non-representative identification/recruitment of subjects
Response	Unrepresentative participation by subjects

Observation bias	
Interviewer	Differential data recording in subject groups by researchers
Recall	Historical data is selectively filtered by subjects

pragmatic trials are a response to the 'diagnostic purity bias' that makes many RCTs unrepresentative. After all, the only entirely representative sample of the whole population of potential subjects is the whole population itself. This is clearly impractical, and is actually less scientifically desirable than a smaller random sample (as there will always be subjects who do not comply with the research and whose absence will introduce 'response bias'). Random samples are those in which every individual in a particular population has an equal chance of being included or excluded. They are practical and desirable, but still susceptible to subject response bias. In practice, however, subjects who do not take part can be usually be replaced by the next subject on the list without introducing significant bias.

The same issues are relevant in enrolling a representative sample of healthy controls in controlled studies. Surveys and cohort studies have the advantage that they can usually identify a representative sample of controls from among the large numbers of non-cases. Randomized controlled trials use the same patients as potential subjects and controls prior to randomization. The problems of recruiting representative controls for other study designs have already been discussed, and recruiting friends and/or relatives is at least acceptable and probably the best available compromise.

Selection biases can be introduced by the researchers (sampling bias) or the subjects (response bias). The common subtypes of **sampling bias** of importance in medical and psychiatric research are 'admission (or Berkson) bias', 'referral filter bias', 'diagnostic purity bias', 'membership bias' and 'historical control bias'. 'Admission (Berkson) bias' has already been discussed in the context of surveys (but applies equally to other descriptive research and case–control studies), and arises where hospitalization rates differ for particular exposure/disease groups, such that the relation between exposure and disease is distorted in hospital-based studies. 'Referral filter bias' occurs when patient referrals from primary to secondary care increase the concentration of rare exposures and severe diseases. This is a well recognized phenomenon in depression. 'Diagnostic purity bias', where the exclusion of comorbidity results in a non-representative sample, is common in RCTs but is a potential problem in all studies. 'Membership bias' is likely where any sort of membership is used to identify subjects, e.g. members of a patients' organization are likely to differ from non-members in a number of ways and hospital staff members are unsuitable controls as they are employed and therefore less likely to have any illness. 'Historical control bias' (just one, but the most important, type of 'non-contemporaneous control bias') arises because secular changes in definitions, exposures, diseases and treatments may render such controls non-comparable. 'Ascertainment bias' results if two groups of subjects are recruited in different ways and differ systematically because of this.

These are all selection biases introduced by the researcher's choice of sampling frame. Random sampling is the best available way of minimizing these problems, but is not foolproof. Even apparently random samples can be biased, e.g. recruiting from the census/voting register/telephone directory excludes those who are not registered because of immigration, poverty, etc. Indeed, if hospitalized patients are the subject group of interest admission bias is unavoidable; and audit studies often have to use patients' past psychiatric histories as their own historical controls. Considering the possibility of sampling bias is therefore required in all research evaluations.

Some selection biases are introduced by the preferential participation or non-participation of different types of research subjects, and can all be thought of as types of **response bias**. 'Non-respondent bias' is the best recognized of these. Non-respondents (and late responders) may exhibit exposures or outcomes that differ from those of respondents (especially early-comers). 'Volunteer bias' is the reverse situation. These can have different effects in medicine and psychiatry. Non-respondents and volunteers in medical studies tend to be healthier than average, whereas in psychiatry the reverse probably applies. This is probably related to the other main type of response bias, 'unacceptable disease bias', i.e. patients with socially stigmatized disorders tend to shy away from researchers (and to underreport their problems). These biases are best reduced by ensuring at least an 80% response rate to surveys (and, by analogy, to all subject recruitment), through the careful initial approach to and resurveying of potential subjects.

To summarize, selection bias is introduced when an individual is identified in such a way that their exposure or disease status is linked to their group status. This is a potential problem for all studies (although least likely in prospective cohort studies). Selection bias can increase or decrease the strength of an association in general, but because of publication bias they are more likely to be found to be increasing false positives. Sampling and response biases in descriptive or case–control studies can sometimes be minimized by good research design and practice, or measured, but this is easier in prospective cohort studies (Sackett 1979). Comparing the summary results of the types of study is often the best measure of bias: if the effects differ in case–control and cohort studies the former are likely to be biased. For example, case–control studies tend to find an increased frequency of obstetric complications in patients with schizophrenia, but cohort studies do not (Geddes & Lawrie 1995).

Observation bias

Observation (measurement or information) bias arises through the systematic and differential misclassification of disease or exposure or both, by researchers (instruments) or subjects. Random or non-differential misclassification, through simply inaccurate information or 'measurement error', is not a bias as such, as it is non-systematic and will only add 'noise' and reduce the strength of any associations. (The only exception to this rule is if there are more than two levels of an exposure, when a false association in one group may be introduced.) Common observation biases of general importance in medical and psychiatric research include interviewer bias, simple attention bias (the Hawthorne effect) and the various sources of recall bias.

Interviewer bias arises when researchers are not blinded to subject status or group membership and (unconsciously or not) tend to alter their approach. If the exposure is measured after the disease this may influence both the intensity and the outcome of a search for exposures in the affected subjects, e.g. by asking more questions ('exposure suspicion bias'). Conversely, 'diagnostic suspicion bias' arises if researchers strive harder to detect disease in those known to have been exposed, or tend to rate outcomes more favourably in the experimental group in an RCT. Generally, all observers (researchers and clinicians) tend to make observations that concur with their expectations ('expectation bias').

These biases will all tend to increase the strength of an association. They can be reduced by the use of highly structured interviews, recording unambiguous information and 'blinding' researchers to group membership – although maintaining blindness can be difficult when exposures, diseases, and especially treatment side-effects are obvious. Employing more than one rater may help and is generally preferable, but also leads to potential problems in establishing interrater reliability (see Chapter 3). The use of self-administered questionnaires (or even computerized assessments) can obviously avoid these difficulties if available (as they are not, for example, in psychosis), but may give rise to subject-based observation biases.

All people tend to alter their behaviour when they know they are being observed – so-called 'attention bias': typically, people tend to normalize their behaviour ('the Hawthorne effect'), which will reduce most associations. If given the opportunity, most people will minimize any perceived deviation from the norm, e.g. reporting less illicit drug use or psychiatric symptoms or family psychiatric history ('social desirability bias'), or simply avoiding the question altogether ('undesirability bias'). These biases will all tend to reduce any differences, but others may not.

Recall bias is a pernicious subject-introduced observation bias, particularly in case–control studies and cross-sectional surveys. Subjects, or informants (relatives), are likely to 'search after meaning' and identify possible exposures. This is also sometimes called 'rumination bias'. For example, depressed patients may be more likely to remember aversive life experiences and mothers of schizophrenics may be more likely to remember obstetric complications ('family information bias'). Conversely, if subjects know they have been exposed they may be more likely to report symptoms of disease. Subjects may also alter responses in the direction they perceive is desired by the investigator ('obsequiousness bias').

Recall biases thereby increase associations in case–control studies. These problems can be minimized by blinding, structured questionnaires/interviews, standardizing the criteria for diseases and exposures, or obtaining corroboratory information from (relatives), case records and databases. Interviews about exposures can also sometimes be conducted before definitive diagnoses are made.

In summary, there are many specific types of bias but they boil down to selection (sampling or response) bias and observation (interviewer or recall) bias. In theory, any bias can increase or decrease the strength of an association, but false positives are more likely in practice (especially if publication bias is allowed for) and observation bias in case–control studies will almost always increase the strength of associations. Cohort studies are inherently less likely to be biased but are more difficult to perform. Selection bias can generally be minimized by careful sampling and subject recruitment, and measurement bias by blind, structured and objective assessments. It is important that studies are designed with these issues in mind, as unlike chance and confounding, bias cannot be evaluated statistically.

Confounding

Confounding is the mixing of effects between an exposure, a disease (or other outcome) and a third factor associated with both, which produces a false association (positive confounding) or obscures a true association (negative confounding). A confounder therefore varies systematically with an exposure *and* acts as (rather than just being associated with) an independent risk or protective factor for the disease. Further, a confounder should be in a triangular relationship with the other variables, rather than on the causal pathway. For example, there is increasing evidence that being born and raised in cities is a risk factor for schizophrenia. If, however, people with schizophrenia tend to 'drift' into cities – as we think they do – the fact that schizophrenia is heritable could account for this association, i.e. a family predisposition to schizophrenia and urban drift could positively confound the (apparent) association between urban upbringing and schizophrenia. Age and sex are common confounders, but can also act as 'effect modifiers'. An effect modifier interacts with an exposure to increase or decrease the risk of disease. For example, depression is most common in middle-aged poor women and may be caused by life events – poverty could confound the association between life events and depression, and age and sex could be effect modifiers.

Confounders can only exert effects if they differ between study groups. Confounding can therefore be reduced by restricting the study population (to the same range of values of a potential confounder), matching (individually, by the frequency of values, or balancing values in the groups) or randomization. Restriction or matching can, however, limit the sample size and possible analysis strategies, resulting in more disadvantageous than beneficial effects: in particular, one cannot study the effect of a matched variable on an outcome. It is generally preferable to include as many subjects as possible to maximize study power, as confounding can then be evaluated and controlled by stratified or multivariate statistical analysis (see Chapter 3). The problem is that it can often be difficult to accurately measure or classify confounders (e.g. genetic liability to schizophrenia). It is therefore better to match for an unquantifiable confounder rather than try to control for it, particularly in small studies, as this will inevitably underadjust for any effect. Attempted statistical control of confounding can therefore leave **residual confounding**. Proxy measures, where a relatively easily measured variable is taken to indicate one that is not available (e.g. paternal social class for childhood environment), are particularly susceptible to this. Residual confounding should therefore always be considered, particularly if an association is reduced after controlling for confounding but some association still remains. On the other hand, confounding can be overcontrolled if two variables are strongly correlated, or if an apparent confounder actually lies on the causal pathway. The problem with the latter is that this interpretation depends upon current biological knowledge. Statistical control for confounding should therefore always present both uncorrected and adjusted values of associations.

One final point needs to be made about confounding. It is obviously true to say that 'one can never exclude a confounder that has not been considered, measured and examined', but the implications of this statement (attributed to Geoffrey Rose) are far-reaching. Basically, you can always wrongfoot a researcher by thinking of a possible confounder that they have not!

REFERENCES AND FURTHER READING

Brugha TS, Lindsay F 1996 Quality of mental health service care: the forgotten pathway from process to outcome. Social Psychiatry and Psychiatric Epidemiology 31: 89–98

Buston K, Parry-Jones W, Livingston M, Bogan A, Wood S 1998 Qualitative research. British Journal of Psychiatry 172: 197–199

Duffy JC, Morrison DP, Peck DF 1998 Research design, measurement and statistics. In: Johnstone EC, Freeman CPL, Zealley AK (eds) Companion to psychiatric studies. Churchill Livingstone, Edinburgh, 149–196

Egger M, Davey Smith G 1998 Meta-analysis: bias in location and selection of studies. British Medical Journal 316: 61–66

Farmer A 1999 The demise of the published case report – is resuscitation necessary? British Journal of Psychiatry 174: 93–94

Geddes JR, Lawrie SM 1995 Obstetric complications and schizophrenia: a meta-analysis. British Journal of Psychiatry 167: 786–790

Grisso JA 1993 Making comparisons. Lancet 342: 157–160

Guyatt G, Sackett D, Taylor DW, Chong J, Roberts R, Pugley S 1986 Determining optimal therapy – randomised trials in individual patients. New England Journal of Medicine 314: 889–892

Hennekens CH, Buring JE 1987 Epidemiology in medicine. Little, Brown & Co, Boston

Hotopf M, Churchill R, Lewis G 1999 Pragmatic randomised controlled trials in psychiatry. British Journal of Psychiatry 175: 217–223

Kernick DP 1998 Economic evaluation in health: a thumbnail sketch. British Medical Journal 316: 1663–1665. [see also the 'economic notes' series throughout 1999 and 2000

Lewis G, Pelosi AJ 1990 The case control study in psychiatry. British Journal of Psychiatry 157: 197–207

Pocock SJ 1983 Clinical trials: a practical approach. John Wiley & Sons, Chichester

Sackett DL 1979 Bias in analytic research. Journal of Chronic Disease 32: 51–63

Sackett DL, Straus SE, Richardson WS, Rosenberg W, Haynes RB 2000 Evidence-based medicine: how to practise and teach EBM, 2nd edition. Churchill-Livingstone, London

Schulz KF, Chalmers I, Hayes RJ, Altman DG 1995 Empirical evidence of bias. Journal of the American Medical Association 273: 408–412

REVISION MCQs

Q1 The following statements are true:

(a) Case report findings can always be attributable to chance
(b) Case series can provide useful information on rare diseases
(c) Studies of disease frequency require a control group
(d) Correlational studies are prone to the ecological fallacy
(e) Qualitative studies do not require a control group

Q2 Case–control studies:

(a) Are prone to bias

(b) Measure the exposure and the disease or outcome retrospectively
(c) Are the optimal research design for rare diseases
(d) Are suitable for the study of rare exposures
(e) Can evaluate multiple outcomes of a single exposure

Q3 Cohort studies:

(a) Require a control group
(b) Are optimal for examining rare exposures
(c) Generally require the disease under study to be common
(d) Demand a short latency between exposure and disease
(e) Are less liable to confounding than case–control studies

Q4 Clinical trials:

(a) Are measures of efficiency
(b) Are most reliable if conducted pragmatically
(c) Require randomized treatment allocation to control for bias
(d) Will overestimate the benefits of experimental treatments without controls
(e) Can deliver reliable results in single subjects

Q5 Systematic reviews:

(a) Have a narrative structure
(b) Can be affected by location bias
(c) Are required before starting any research project
(d) Can be reliably done by a single researcher
(e) Do not require statistical analysis

Q6 Meta-analysis:

(a) Of randomized controlled trials provides the best evidence of whether a treatment works
(b) Is unreliable unless based on a systematic review
(c) Is most reliable if based on dichotomous outcomes
(d) Of observational studies is less reliable than meta-analysis of experimental studies
(e) Is sensitive to publication bias

Q7 The following are potential explanations of an association:

(a) Random error
(b) Bias
(c) Cause
(d) Residual confounding
(e) Reverse causality

Q8 The following observations increase the chance that an observed association is true:

(a) Strength of the association
(b) Specificity
(c) Temporal sequence
(d) Consistency
(e) Plausibility

Q9 Bias:

(a) Is possible in any study
(b) Is unlikely in clinical trials
(c) Can be avoided
(d) Can be measured and controlled for statistically
(e) Can be introduced into a study by researchers or subjects

Q10 A confounder:

(a) Is associated with both an exposure and a disease
(b) Is on the causal pathway between exposure and disease
(c) Is always a risk or protective factor for the disease in question
(d) Can be controlled for in the design stage of a study
(e) Can be controlled for statistically

ANSWERS

A1

(a) True
(b) True
(c) False
(d) True
(e) True

A2

(a) True
(b) True (unless they are prospective, which is very rare)
(c) True
(d) False (this is true of cohort studies)
(e) False (this is true of cohort studies)

A3

(a) False (studies of prognosis do not have to be controlled)
(b) True
(c) True
(d) False (this is preferable but not essential)
(e) False (bias is more likely in case–control studies, but both are liable to confounding)

A4

(a) False (trials measure efficacy/effectiveness)
(b) False (RCTs are reliable, pragmatic trials are generalizable)
(c) False (randomization controls for confounding, bias can still be a problem)
(d) True
(e) True

A5

(a) False
(b) True
(c) True
(d) False (study selection and data acquisition need to be checked with another researcher)
(e) True

A6

(a) True (unless a well-conducted mega-trial is available)
(b) True
(c) True (as all data can therefore be included)
(d) True
(e) True

A7

(a) True
(b) True
(c) True
(d) True
(e) True (although this is not possible in prospective cohort studies)

A8

(a) True
(b) True (this was originally included as a criterion of causality, as was reversibility in an RCT, but later seen as excessive as many exposures may have different eventualities depending on host factors and other exposures)
(c) True
(d) True
(e) True

A9

(a) True
(b) False (observer bias is possible)
(c) False (although it can be reduced)
(d) False (this is only true of confounding)
(e) True

A10

(a) True
(b) False
(c) True
(d) True
(e) True

3

Statistics

Mention of statistics is often enough to cause an involuntary shutdown of doctors' minds, a response conditioned by badly presented and seemingly irrelevant lectures in undergraduate years and reinforced by a general avoidance of numbers in medical training. This is a cause for concern as well as a great shame. An innumerate doctor is a potentially dangerous one and statistics can provide certainty, or at least consensus, when various pieces of information are contradictory. Indeed, conducting statistical analyses of research data and suddenly appreciating the (sometimes wonderfully simple) mathematics of and interrelationships between statistical tests is both stimulating and rewarding.

The central problem with texts on medical statistics is that they often appear to be written by people who are more conscious of the rules governing the application of various tests than how innumerate the average doctor really is. There are several notable exceptions, some of which we will refer to in this chapter (e.g. Gardner & Altman 1989, Swinscow 1996), but only one written specifically for psychiatrists (Duffy et al 1998). We take the view that statistics are tools to help make sense of data, rather than rules to follow slavishly, and that it is possible to present the main concepts in everyday prose. We do, however, think that an acquaintance with the mathematics of statistics helps to understand them, and therefore present some of the main formulae in this chapter, although we do not expect the reader to memorize them. Although it is true that one needs to analyse one's own data before one can truly appreciate the use of many statistical tests, and that detailed statistical knowledge takes years to acquire, it is possible very quickly to understand the meaning and accurate application of many terms and tests. Indeed, this is the minimum required to be able to appraise the use of statistics in any published paper.

In the syllabus for the MRCPsych several specific tests are mentioned as topics that trainees are expected to know about.

These include the application of the *t*-test, analysis of variance, the chi-squared (χ^2) test, odds ratios, multiple regression, logistic regression and confidence intervals, as well as an awareness of the differences between probability, statistical significance and clinical significance. Although we are fortunate to have a definite syllabus, this list does not include tests and concepts that are just as important and actually help to provide an integrated understanding of medical statistics. We aim to provide such an understanding in this chapter, and are therefore more inclusive than the exam syllabus. The exam syllabus also mentions a number of statistics that have been specifically devised to aid critical appraisal. These are therefore discussed in the next chapter (i.e. sensitivity, specificity and the likelihood ratio in the section on diagnosis; and the absolute and relative risk reduction and the number needed to treat in treatment).

We therefore trust that what follows is comprehensible and comprehensive. We will start by considering the types of data generated in medical research, then deal with basic descriptive and inferential (comparative) statistics, various measures of association, multivariate statistical tests (which look at several variables simultaneously) and the main statistical considerations in meta-analysis. As in the previous chapter, psychiatric examples will be used wherever possible.

TYPES OF DATA

Any data from scientific measurement are either continuous (dimensional) or categorical (discrete). Continuous or dimensional data can have any value within the range of all possible values (e.g. age and height). Categorical or discrete data, on the other hand, can only have set values (of whole numbers) and can be usefully subdivided as follows:

- Binary data – where there are only two mutually exclusive categories (e.g. ill/not, dead/alive)
- Nominal data – where three or more unique categories bear no mathematical relation to each other (e.g. qualitative data such as marital status coded numerically for analysis)
- Ordinal data – where, in addition, there is an order inherent in the measurement scale but this is not simply quantifiable (e.g. social classes I–V, where the difference between I and II

cannot be said to be the same as the difference between IV and V)
* Interval data – where the order is meaningful in that differences between the points are equal across the scale, but zero is just a point on the scale without representing an absence of the characteristic (e.g. the Farenheit scale of temperature)
* Ratio data – where, in addition, the scale has a true zero (e.g. degrees Celsius and the scores on most symptom rating scales).

The importance of these distinctions is in the types of statistical test that can be applied to the different types of data. Technically, other factors are also important in choosing the correct test, but in practice the type and distribution of data are by far the most important. Most continuous measures, ratio and interval data are approximately normally distributed and can therefore be analysed with parametric statistics, using the mean and standard deviation. Ordinal (or ranked) data are not normally distributed and must be analysed with non-parametric statistics, using the median and range. Binary/nominal data can only be compared in terms of the modal values and frequency counts. However, binary data probably have inherently greater clinical value, and can easily be transformed into a single comparative measure (e.g. an odds ratio) that has many useful statistical properties (e.g. for meta-analysis; see p. 80).

RATIOS

A ratio is probably the most basic unit of descriptive statistics, as it simply describes the relationship between two numbers (note that this is not the same as the ratio data mentioned above). This has some valuable uses, especially in quantifying disease frequencies and mortalities.

A **ratio** is expressed as the relationship between the numerator and the denominator, the instances of an observation in any reference group, and can have any value between zero and infinity. A **proportion** is a special type of ratio in which the numerator is included in the denominator, and can therefore be expressed as a percentage, ranging from 0 to 100%. A **rate** is a ratio that is, or should be, quoted with reference to a time frame, i.e. the number of events relative to a standard frequency measurement, such as per person-year. It should, however, be noted that doctors tend to use these terms very loosely. As it is illogical and often misleading to compare two different measures, one should always check how any reported ratio measure is defined and calculated (Hennekens & Buring 1987).

There are two main **measures of disease frequency** – prevalence and incidence. The prevalence is the number of individuals with a disease in a population at a particular point in time (**point prevalence**) or over a period of time (**period prevalence**). Note that the former is a proportion and the latter is a rate (even if the distinction between a point and a period is rather arbitrary). The period prevalence rate is sometimes used in psychiatry, as many disorders have a time criterion of weeks or months in their definition, although it has the disadvantage that it combines prevalent and incident cases in one measure.

The incidence (or inception) is the number of new cases of a disease over a period of time out of the total population at risk (the **incidence risk** or **cumulative incidence**), or out of the total person-time of observation (the **incidence rate** or **incidence density**). The reason for the distinction is that the numbers at risk of developing a disease may change over time, through death or loss to follow-up, such that the incidence risk/cumulative incidence can be unreliable. The incidence rate/density explicitly allows for this, as individuals can provide varying person-years of observation. For example, a subject followed for 5 years provides 5 person-years' observation, as do five subjects followed for only a year. This means that the incidence rate can be more reliably used to quantify the risk of development of a disorder over a certain period of time. The **lifetime risk**, also known as the morbid risk or expectancy, is a type of incidence risk as it describes the number of cases in a population over the length of an average lifetime.

It is worth noting that the prevalence is proportional to the product of the incidence rate and average duration of a disease. Indeed, if the incidence rate and duration are stable and the prevalence is low, the prevalence is equal to the product of the two. It is therefore possible that a disease can have a high prevalence, despite a low incidence, if the duration is long.

The **mortality rate** is a type of incidence rate that expresses the risk of death in a population over a time period. These can be quoted as 'crude rates' or as 'category-specific rates' (e.g. age-specific mortality gives the death rate in the population in that age range). It is, however, often useful to have a single measure of mortality for a population which allows for the make-up of that population, so that different populations can be compared on one rather than several measures. This is done by taking a 'weighted' average of category-specific rates, in a process called adjustment or standardization. For example, the **standardized mortality ratio (SMR)** is calculated as the ratio of observed to expected deaths, the latter being obtained by multiplying ('weighting') the category-specific rates by the number of person-years of observation in each category and then adding them all together.

All of these ratios are ratio measures, and can therefore be analysed with parametric or non-parametric statistics as appropriate to their distribution.

DESCRIPTIVE STATISTICS – MEASURES OF CENTRAL TENDENCY AND DISPERSION

The usual first step in any statistical analysis is to examine and describe the data. The distribution of values should be examined to identify any mistyped values or outliers, and to determine whether parametric or non-parametric descriptives and tests should be used. Data with a normal (gaussian) distribution ('the bell-shaped curve'; Figure 3.1), or data that can be made normally

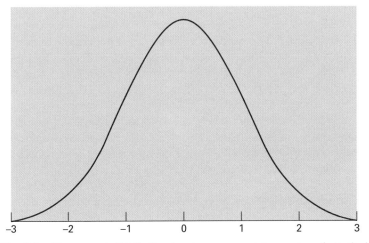

Fig. 3.1 The normal distribution (numbers represent the number of standard deviations from the mean).

distributed by, for example, log transformation, are best described by the **mean** (the sum of all values divided by the number of values) and the **standard deviation** (the spread of all observations around the mean, calculated as the square root of the variance).

The **variance** is the sum of all the differences between all the values and the mean, squared (so that negative and positive deviations do not cancel out) and divided by the total number of observations minus 1 (the 'degrees of freedom'). The degrees of freedom is so-called and calculated because there is that number $(n - 1)$ of independent differences between the observations in a sample. Note that approximately 68% of all the data will be within one standard deviation above and below the mean, and approximately 95% will be within 1.96 (approximately 2) standard deviations of the mean.

$$\text{Mean or } \bar{x} = \frac{\sum x}{n}$$

$$\text{Standard deviation (SD)} = \sqrt{Variance} = \sqrt{\frac{\sum (x - \bar{x})^2}{n - 1}}$$

Ordinal, ratio and continuous data which are 'skewed' (where the most common values are off to the left or right of the distribution) or 'bimodal' (with two peaks) need to be described by the median and the (interquartile) range. In these cases the mean is unreliable, as it is disproportionately influenced by extreme values (outliers). The **median** is the central value, in the middle of all the values; the **interquartile range** is the difference between the values that are midway between the median and the two extremes; the **range** is the difference between the lowest and highest values. The median and interquartile range are simply calculated if there is an odd number of values, and if there is an even number of values the average of the two nearest values is taken. Note that the median gives no information about the data distribution, whereas the mean does.

As already stated, binary/nominal data can only be described by the **mode**, the most common value, and the frequencies of certain values (as a proportion of the total).

Examples
In the normally distributed data set 1,2,2,3,3,3,4,4,5

$$\text{mean} = 3, \text{median} = 3, \text{mode} = 3$$
$$\text{standard deviation} = \sqrt{(4+1+1+0+0+0+1+1+4)/8} = 1.2$$
$$\text{range} = 1 \text{ to } 5 = 4$$

Note that the mean, median and mode are all the same in normally distributed data.

In the non-gaussian data set 5,10,15,20,100

mean = 30, but the median = 15 (interquartile range = 10–20 or 10)

CONFIDENCE INTERVAL

The confidence interval (CI), or confidence limits, is a special measure of the dispersion of data with properties that bridge the gap between descriptive and analytical statistics. The CI gives the precision of a measure, as any measure from any sample data set can only be regarded as an estimate of the true situation in the population as a whole. The CI can be defined as the range within which the true measure actually lies, with a specific degree of assurance (usually 95%), based upon the estimate from your data set (Gardner & Altman 1989). In other words, one can be 95% certain that the true population value of a measure (a proportion, mean, etc.) is within the 95%CI, or between the two confidence limits of your estimate.

Confidence limits are most accurately found by consulting scientific tables. They can be calculated approximately but relatively simply as the measure plus or minus 1.96 (approximately 2) times the standard error of the measure, although the formulae for standard errors depend on the measure of interest. The **standard error** (SE) uses the variability of the sample measure as an estimate of the true effect in the general population from which the sample was drawn. In other words, the SE reflects how much the mean and standard deviation would be likely to vary in other samples from the same population. For example, the mean plus or minus the standard error gives 68% of the values in the general population. We give the formulae for the SE and CI for a mean and a proportion here and others below as appropriate.

CI for a population mean $\approx$ mean $\pm 1.96 \times$ SE

$$\text{SE (of a mean)} = \frac{\text{SD}}{\sqrt{n}}$$

e.g. from above, mean = 3, SD = 1.2, n = 9; then SE = 1.2/3 = 0.4, 95%CI ≈ 2.2–3.8.

CI for a proportion (as a decimal)

$$\text{SE (of a proportion '}p\text{')} = \sqrt{\frac{p(1-p)}{n}}$$

e.g. if p = 0.5, n = 100; then SE = $\sqrt{0.25/100}$ = 0.05, 95%CI ≈ 0.4–0.6.

It is readily apparent from these formulae that the size of the sample (n) is a major determinant of the SE and hence the 'width' of the CI. If, for example, the mean had been estimated in a sample of 100, the 95%CI would be 2.8–3.2. The larger the sample, the more likely the results are true, i.e. the narrower the CI, the more confidence one can have in the results. This alludes to one of the major values of the CI when it comes to analytical statistics or hypothesis testing.

The confidence interval is related to probability – it is no accident that the usual values are 95% and 5%, respectively – but more informative. The CI gives all the information of a P value plus the precision of any estimate. A narrow confidence interval means little variability in the estimate of the effect owing to large sample size. This is particularly useful when interpreting data that are not statistically significant. For example, if the 95%CI of a difference between the means in two groups overlaps with zero (no difference), then the corresponding P value is by definition greater than 0.05. If the 95%CI in this example was narrow, then we could have greater faith that this was a true negative finding. If the confidence interval was wide, however, the data would be compatible with a real difference but the sample size was not sufficient to have adequate power to exclude chance as an explanation of the findings (see below).

PROBABILITY, STATISTICAL SIGNIFICANCE AND CLINICAL SIGNIFICANCE

Probability (P) simply refers to the likelihood of any event occurring relative to (i.e. as a proportion of) the total number of possibilities, e.g. the chance of throwing any number on a die is one-out-of-six or 1/6 or 0.17 or 17%.

Statistical significance is arbitrarily assigned to events which would have occurred by chance alone less than once in 20 times, i.e. less than 5% of the time, or $P<0.05$. Put another way, any statistical test has a 1/20 chance of being statistically significant by chance alone, i.e. any data set subjected to a 'data dredging' should yield at least one 'significant result' at $P<0.05$ for every 20 (two-tailed) significance tests. **Two-tailed** refers to the two tails of the data distribution, i.e. any group measure is simultaneously tested to be smaller or larger than another group. This is the usual method of statistical testing. Occasionally, one comes across **one-tailed** tests of a very specific hypothesis, but these are very rarely justified and should arouse suspicion. If only one side of the data distribution is examined (in essence stating that the opposite result is inconceivable), the probability of any eventuality is thereby doubled and $P<0.1$ is effectively adopted as statistically significant.

Statistical significance is, however, very different from **clinical significance** (which is one of the main reasons for the statistics of evidence-based medicine described in the next chapter). Statistical tests are generally very sensitive to the sample size, so that if one uses a large enough number of subjects even a small difference between groups will be statistically significant. Similarly, a statistically significant difference in, for example, means does not necessarily tell one very much about the value of such a measure in discriminating between two populations, for example, healthy and diseased. Ideally, members of two such populations will have mean values that do not overlap, i.e. the measure has a bimodal distribution, but this is very rare in clinical practice. For example, most blood test reference values are calculated from a (local) population mean plus/minus two standard deviations, so that 1/20 blood tests will be abnormal by chance alone and any values just outside the 'normal range' may not be clinically significant.

In summary, a P value of less than 0.05 is an inferential aid that does not in itself quantify the extent of the difference, because of the importance of the 'degrees of freedom' ($n - 1$) in any comparison. This is why the 95%CI is so useful.

TYPES I AND II ERRORS, EFFECT SIZES AND POWER CALCULATIONS

Type I errors occur when the null hypothesis, i.e. that there is no difference between two groups, is rejected when it is in fact true (i.e. a false positive). This can arise for any number of reasons, such as bias in measurements or confounding between measures. Statistically, the probability of making a type I error is equal to the P value and is expressed as α. For example, an α of 0.05 means that there is (only) a 5% chance of erroneously rejecting the null hypothesis.

Type II errors occur when the null hypothesis is accepted when it is in fact false (i.e. a false negative). This usually occurs when a real difference between groups is obscured by a small sample size and/or a large variance (from, for example, measurement noise or error). The probability of making a type II error is represented by β.

The **power** of a study is defined as the probability of (correctly) rejecting the null hypothesis when a true difference exists, and is represented as $1-\beta$. Typically, β is arbitrarily set at 0.2. Thus, a typical study has 0.8 of a chance or 80% power to detect a specified degree of difference (the effect size) at a specified degree of significance.

Effect sizes are simply calculated as the difference between two means divided by the standard deviation in controls (or the average of two standard deviations in two patient groups). The former is sometimes called 'Cohen's d' and the latter the 'standardized difference'. These are also numerically equivalent to 'z scores'. Ideally, effect sizes should be calculated from a small pilot study of the proposed study, which will also reveal any difficulties in the means of recruitment or measurement. Pilot studies may not always be practical, however, in which case typical effect sizes from similar previous studies can sometimes be calculated.

A power calculation allows one to estimate the numbers of subjects in two groups required to render a difference statistically significant. For example, if a randomized controlled trial expected mean outcome scores of 4 and 2, with an averaged (or 'pooled') standard deviation of 2, with α set at 0.05 and β at 0.2:

$$\text{group } n = \frac{2 \times \text{SD}^2}{(\text{difference in means})^2} \times f(\alpha,\beta)$$

$\qquad$ = 8/4 × ~8 [the factorial value of $f(\alpha,\beta)$ – see Pocock 1983]

$\qquad$ = ~16 patients in each arm of the trial.

This is a typical trial size in psychiatry, but is for a relatively large effect size of 1 (2/2) and would still have a 1/5 chance of failing to find a true difference. A lack of power must always therefore be considered as a possible explanation for a 'negative trial', or indeed any negative finding. Note that there are a number of resources available for determining the numbers required in a study without actually having to do the calculation: Gore & Altman (1982) give a nomogram, and several statistical packages are available (see Resources, p. 84).

There are different power formulae for qualitative and quantitative outcome measures and for situations where treatment equivalence is sought. The latter usually requires hundreds of patients in each treatment arm. Thus, the commonly encountered phrase in the drug industry literature that a new drug is 'as least as effective as' a standard treatment is usually incorrect, as failing to find a difference (through low power, for example) is not the same as demonstrating equivalence.

ANALYTICAL STATISTICS

In statistical analyses we are generally interested in comparing two or more groups of observations. Ideally, measurements have been made to test a particular hypothesis about putative differences between groups. Following Karl Popper, hypotheses should be stated as null hypotheses (i.e. that there is no difference) and statistical tests are used to attempt to refute the null hypothesis (i.e. to show that there is *not* no difference). This is because, philosophically, one cannot prove anything from empirical observation, but one can disprove falsities, i.e. identifying the truth is actually achieved by moving further away from error, rather than discovering truth.

It should be noted here, however, that there are alternatives to this rather limited view of scientific endeavour, that of Bayesian statistics. The latter builds upon all available information in the light of new findings, to give a measure of the likelihood of interpretations. This is an increasingly popular approach to medical statistics, particularly in evidence-based medicine, which finds an obvious use in the likelihood ratios used in considering the value of diagnostic tests (see Chapter 4), but is not as yet mainstream and is not therefore considered further here.

Returning to analytical statistics, there are a small number of regularly used tests which apply to particular situations, depending on the type of data, the number of groups being compared and the characteristics of the groups. These are shown in Table 3.1 and will now be discussed in turn.

Table 3.1 Commonly used statistical tests

	Parametric	Non-parametric	Binary
Descriptive	Mean, standard deviation	Median, interquartile range	Mode, frequencies
Comparing 2 groups			
independent	Student's independent *t* test	Mann–Whitney U test	χ^2 test
paired	Student's paired *t* test	Wilcoxon's rank sum test	McNemar test
Comparing >2 groups	Analysis of variance (ANOVA)	Kruskal–Wallis ANOVA	χ^2 test

DIFFERENCES IN MEANS – THE *t* STATISTIC

With data that are approximately normally distributed the means in two groups are compared with **Student's *t* test** (an independent *t* test if the two groups are different subjects, a paired *t* test if they are the same subjects at different time points). The value of the ***t* statistic** is calculated as the difference between the means divided by the standard error of the difference in means (calculated from the pooled SD):

$$t = \frac{\bar{x}_1 - \bar{x}_2}{\sqrt{\dfrac{SD_1^2}{n_1} + \dfrac{SD_2^2}{n_2}}}$$

Note that the *t* test assumes that the variance of the data in the two groups is more or less equal. If this is not the case – as a rough rule of thumb, the standard deviations differ by a factor of more than 2 – then a slightly modified equation applies. The *t* statistic is also calculated slightly differently if the groups are paired, or matched on important variables, but the formulae still amount to dividing the difference in means by the standard error of that difference.

The statistical significance of the *t* value is found from tables of the *t* distribution (e.g. Swinscow 1996, p. 134), allowing for the degrees of freedom (df) (the number of observations minus 1, for both groups, i.e. $n - 2$). The example below is an edited printout from the Statistical Package for the Social Science (SPSS) applied to one of our data sets; this is one of the most widely used software applications for statistics in medicine.

Example of a t test (for independent samples) printout from SPSS applied to one of our data sets

Variable 'X'	n of cases	Mean	SD	SE of mean
Group 1	30	12.7333	4.586	0.837
Group 2	14	18.5714	3.056	0.817

Mean difference = –5.8381;
Levene's test for equality of variances: $F = 2.615$, $P = 0.113$

t test for equality of means:

Variances	t value	df	2-tail sig.	SE of diff.	95%CI for diff.
Equal	–4.32	42	0.000	1.351	(–8.564, –3.112)
Unequal	–4.99	36.57	0.000	1.170	(–8.209, –3.467)

The non-significant value of Levene's test (see SPSS manuals) shows that the variances are sufficiently similar to use the equal variances *t* test. The *P* value is quoted as '0.000', but this means that $P<0.001$ as $P = 0$ is not possible. The 95%CI is (approximately) equal to the mean difference (diff.) plus or minus 1.96 times the standard error of the difference in means.

DIFFERENCES IN MEANS – THE *F* STATISTIC

With normally distributed data in three or more groups, the appropriate test is an analysis of variance (ANOVA). One-way ANOVA is suitable for independent measures, repeated measures ANOVA for measures taken on two or more occasions in the same groups of individuals. In any ANOVA the variability between the group means is compared with the variability of observations around the mean within the groups. The ratio of the former to the latter is the *F* **statistic**.

Between-groups variability is calculated as the sum of all the differences between each group mean from the overall mean, squared and multiplied by the number of observations in that group:

$$n_1(\bar{x}_1 - \bar{x}_{\text{total}})^2 + n_2(\bar{x}_2 - \bar{x}_{\text{total}})^2 + n_3(\bar{x}_3 - \bar{x}_{\text{total}})^2 \ldots$$

This sum of squares is divided by the appropriate degrees of freedom (the number of groups minus 1) to give the 'mean sum of squares' between groups.

Within-groups variability is calculated by multiplying each of the group variances (V, the square of each standard deviation) by the number of cases in the group minus 1 and then adding up the results:

$$(n_1 - 1)V_1 + (n_2 - 1)V_2 + (n_3 - 1)V_3 \ldots$$

This sum of squares is divided by the appropriate degrees of freedom (the number of observations minus the number of groups) to give the mean sum of squares within groups.

If the null hypothesis is true the between-groups mean square and the within-groups mean square should be close to each other, and one divided by the other (the F value) will be close to 1. Once again, the statistical significance of this value is consulted from tables of the F distribution, according to the degrees of freedom (the number of observations minus 1).

Note that ANOVA only tells you if there are significant differences between the groups, rather than where the differences are. To identify which groups differ from the others, one of the **post hoc significance tests** is required. The simplest approach is to do multiple t tests between all pairs of group means, in a 'least significant difference' test, but such multiple comparisons are prone to finding differences by chance alone. One alternative is to use a **Bonferroni correction**, which divides the significance level by the number of observations (e.g. if five comparisons are being made the observed P value must be less than 0.05/5 or 0.01 to be significant at the 0.05 level), but this is generally regarded as too stringent. The post hoc 'Scheffe test' or 'Tukey's honestly significant difference test' offer a suitable compromise as they control for multiple comparisons without being too conservative.

Example of an ANOVA SPSS printout from one of our data sets
Variable 'Y'
By variable group

Source	df	Sum of squares	Mean squares	F ratio	F prob.
Between-groups	2	800.9833	400.4917	3.4494	0.0385
Within-groups	57	6618.0000	116.1053		
Total	59	7418.9833			

Group	Count	Mean	Standard Deviation	Standard Error	95% CI for mean
1	30	51.2667	10.4977	1.9166	47.3468–55.1866
2	15	46.2000	13.2298	3.4159	38.8736–53.5264
3	15	56.5333	8.3312	2.1511	51.9196–61.1470
Total	60	51.3167	11.2136	1.4477	48.4199–54.2135

NON-PARAMETRIC COMPARISONS

For non-normally distributed variables, non-parametric statistics should be employed. The three commonly used tests (see Table 3.1) all adopt essentially the same approach – indeed, the Mann–Whitney and Wilcoxon tests have been shown to be the same. The data are ranked or ordered, the ranks are then summed for each group, and the lowest total rank is compared with tables of ranks and corresponding probability values (see Swinscow 1996 and SPSS manuals for further details). Thus, technically, ranks rather than medians are compared – it is possible to have groups with similar medians who differ significantly on ranks.

By convention, the Wilcoxon rank sum test is used for paired data, the Mann–Whitney for two independent groups, and the Kruskal–Wallis for three or more groups. There are no post hoc non-parametric tests: if the Kruskal–Wallis finds an overall difference, post hoc Mann–Whitney tests must be done.

Note that these tests can be used to compare parametric data, but parametric testing is more powerful, makes the calculation of confidence intervals easier and is more flexible when one wants to examine the interrelationships of more than two variables, e.g. examining for possible confounding in multivariate statistics.

DIFFERENCES IN PROPORTIONS

Two proportions of discontinuous variables, from two or more independent samples, must be compared using the **chi-square test** (χ^2). This is concerned with the difference between actual observed values and what would be expected if the values followed the same proportions as the total number of observations. Mathematically, this is expressed as:

$$\chi^2 = \frac{(O_1 - E_1)^2}{E_1} + \frac{(O_2 - E_2)^2}{E_2} + \dots$$

The value of χ^2 is then compared with the distribution (see, for example, Swinscow 1996, p. 135), according to the appropriate number of degrees of freedom (the number of columns minus 1 multiplied by the numbers of rows minus 1).

Example of a χ^2 test SPSS printout (adapted) from one of our data sets

Group by sex

	Sex Observed count Expected value		Row total
Group 1	11 10.0	19 20.0	30 50.0%
Group 2	5 5.0	10 10.0	15 25.0%
Group 3	4 5.0	11 10.0	15 25.0%
Column	20	40	60
Total	33.3%	66.7%	100.0%

χ^2	Value	df	Significance
Pearson	0.45000	2	0.79852

In this example, Pearson's $\chi^2 = (11 - 10)^2/10 + (19 - 20)^2/20 + (5 - 5)^2/5 + (10 - 10)^2/10 + (4 - 5)^2/5 + (11 - 10)^2/10 = 0.1 + 0.05 + 0 + 0 + 0.2 + 0.1 = 0.45$.

If this P value were significant one would have to do tests between each of the pairs of groups to find where the differences were. This is sometimes referred to as splitting the χ^2 table, i.e. into a series of '2 × 2' or 'contingency' tables (Table 3.2). Such contingency tables have found many applications in medical statistics (e.g. odds ratios), as we shall see below. Of particular note is that any χ^2 analysis can be broken down by other variables (e.g. age groups) to see if there are any subgroup differences in the original measures. This is called 'a stratified analysis' and is the essence of multivariate statistics.

This flexibility of the χ^2 test comes at a price: it is very sensitive to sample size. It used to be said that a **Yates correction** should be applied if the total sample was less than 100 or any cell value was less than 10, and that **Fisher's exact probability test** should be used if any cell value was less than 5, but both these qualifications are probably too stringent (see SPSS manuals). χ^2 tests must always be applied to the original data, not, for example, to percentages, which would inflate any differences. Finally, there is a special type of χ^2 test for matched data – the **McNemar test** – which is calculated differently (see Swinscow 1996).

Table 3.2   Example of a 2 × 2 table

	Outcome yes	Outcome no	
Exposed – yes	a	b	a + b
Exposed – no	c	d	c + d
	a + c	b + d	a + b + c + d (n)

MEASURES OF ASSOCIATION

When comparing two groups it is often possible to express any differences between them with a single measure – the association between them. Common examples include the relative (ratio) measures expressed in odds ratios, relative risks, and correlation and regression, which we will discuss in detail below. There are also other important measures of association, which we will now briefly discuss.

The simplest measure is that of **agreement** or **concordance**, i.e. the extent to which two measures come to exactly the same conclusion as a proportion of all measures. In a standard two-by-two table (see Table 3.2), where the rows and columns would represent whether each measure or rater found a phenomenon or not, this is calculated as a + d/n. This statistic is sometimes presented as a measure of the reliability of a research assessment, but does not allow for the fact that some agreement will occur by chance alone. Chance agreement is allowed for in the calculation of (Cohen's) **kappa** (κ), by comparing the actual and potential agreement beyond chance, expressed as a fraction between 0 and 1 (see Sackett et al 1991, pp 28–31 for details). However, κ is sensitive to the base rate, i.e. if the prevalence is <20% or >80%, κ will rarely be above 0.3.

The **reliability** of a measure is the extent to which that measure is stable between raters (interrater reliability), within one rater over time (intrarater reliability), between two halves of a scale (split-half scale reliability), or between all the items in a scale (internal consistency). Reliability can be quantified as a correlation coefficient or (where more than two raters are evaluated) the intraclass correlation coefficient (ICC). Plain correlations are, however, insensitive to consistent differences between raters, and the ICC can be calculated by many (often inconsistent) methods. It may therefore be best to calculate the mean difference between raters and the standard deviation of that mean (Bland & Altman 1986). Simple correlations are, however, a satisfactory measure of the reliability of a scale, whether these are calculated as the correlation between the two halves ('split-half coefficients') or as the average of all the correlations between the items ('Cronbach's α').

Validity is a related but distinct concept: the extent to which a measure actually measures what it purports to, which is quantified as above. There are many subtypes: face validity (simply appearing to be valid); concurrent (compared with an alternative measure of the same thing); predictive or construct (accurately predicting the future); and content or sampling validity (the completeness of assessment of the phenomenon).

ODDS RATIOS

An odds ratio is a measure of the strength of an association, calculated by comparing outcomes in exposed and non-exposed persons. In a case–control study the exposure is often the presence or absence of a risk factor for a disease, and the outcome is the presence or absence of the disease. In a controlled trial the exposures will be the new or experimental treatment and the old or placebo treatment, with the outcome being any clinically relevant dichotomous measure.

It is important to understand the difference and relationship between odds and probability. In throwing a die, for example, the probability (P) of any number coming up is one-out-of-six, or 1/6 (see above), whereas the odds (O) of any number is one-to-five, or 1/5, i.e. the denominator includes the primary observation in the former but not the latter. Thus,

$$P = \frac{O}{O+1} \text{ and } O = \frac{P}{1-P}$$

Comparing the odds in the two subject groups, as 'relative odds' or 'ratios of the odds', gives an odds ratio (OR). An OR of 1.0 (or 'unity') therefore reflects exactly the same outcome proportions in both groups, i.e. no effect. The odds ratio is calculated as (see Table 3.2 for notation) the odds of exposure among the cases (a/c) relative to or divided by that in controls (b/d), i.e. (a/c)/(b/d). As dividing by a fraction is equivalent to multiplying by its reciprocal:

$$OR = \frac{ab}{bc}$$

Example

Imagine that a new drug is being evaluated against an old drug in terms of the likelihood of bringing about some measure of clinical improvement, in a trial of 100 subjects with 50 in each group. The hypothetical results of 40 improved subjects on the new drug and 30 on the old drug can be represented in a contingency table as below (Table 3.3).

Table 3.3 Hypothetical treatment trial results

	Improved	Not improved	
New drug	40	10	50
Old drug	30	20	50
Total	70	30	100

The odds of improvement are therefore 40/10 and 30/20, respectively. The OR of improving is (40/10)/(30/20) or (40 × 20)/(30 × 10) = 800/300 = 2.67. Thus patients receiving the new treatment are on average 2.67 times more likely to improve than not, compared with those getting the old treatment. Note that this could equally be phrased as patients getting the old treatment are 300/800 or 1/ 2.67 or 0.375 times less likely to improve. This 'reciprocity' is one of the important mathematical properties of the odds ratio, another being that it is a useful measure for comparing studies in a meta-analysis. The fact that one needs dichotomous or binary data to calculate an odds ratio is another argument for using such measures in a clinical trial, as well as that dichotomous outcomes are probably more clinically relevant in general.

The **relative risk** (RR) is a similar statistic, as applied to cohort studies, which is calculated as the ratio of the disease or outcome in the exposed (a/a + b) to that in the non-exposed (c/c + d):

$$RR = \frac{a/(a+b)}{c/(c+d)} = \frac{ac+ad}{ac+bc}$$

As these expressions include the denominator, the RR is generally a more reliable statistic than the OR. As with all contingency table data the OR is sensitive to relatively small changes in assigning outcomes to cases as introduced by misclassification bias and other biases. Generally the OR will be higher than the RR, sometimes by as much as a factor. Note, however, that the OR approximates to the RR if the disease or outcome is rare ('the rare disease assumption'), as the 'ac' product in both numerator and denominator cancels out (see Hennekens & Buring 1987 for further details).

As odds ratios and relative risks can only vary between zero and infinity, the calculation of their confidence intervals requires the use of logarithms (akin to logarithmic transformation for skewed data) and antilogarithms. The basic formula for a 95%CI remains, but this must be calculated by adding and subtracting 1.96 times the natural log of the standard error to the natural log of the OR before antilogarithm conversion:

95%CI of OR $\approx$ antilog [($\log_e$ OR) $\pm$ (1.96 $\times$ $\log_e$ SE)]

the natural log of the standard error of an OR being $\sqrt{(1/a + 1/b + 1/c + 1/d)}$.

The (various) formulae for calculating the 95%CI for a relative risk are given in Hennekens & Buring (1987), for example. If the 95%CI of an OR or RR includes 1.0 (unity), then the corresponding P value is by definition greater than 0.05. As before, however, the confidence interval gives information on the precision of this estimate, such that if the 95%CI is narrow we can have greater faith that this is a true negative, whereas if the confidence interval is wide the data are compatible with a true increased/decreased risk.

The OR and RR are relative measures of association, but absolute measures can be useful. The **attributable risk** (AR) or 'risk difference' is simply the difference in disease (outcome) proportions in the exposed and non-exposed groups. This therefore quantifies the risk attached to the exposure of interest, with the effect of any other factors removed, i.e. the number of cases of disease among the exposed that can be attributed to the exposure. This is clearly related to the number of cases of the *disease in the exposed* that could be eliminated if the exposure were eliminated (assuming the exposure is causal). This **attributable proportion** (or fraction) is the AR divided by the rate of disease among the exposed and is usually expressed as a percentage. The AR can also be extrapolated to estimate the number of cases of a *disease in the general population* that could be eliminated if the exposure were eliminated. The **population attributable fraction** (or **risk** or **rate**) is the product of the AR and the proportion of exposed individuals in the population. Note that these calculations use incidence rates from cohort studies, but that different equations can be used in case–control studies (see Hennekens & Buring 1987).

CORRELATION AND REGRESSION

A correlation (study or coefficient) measures the degree of association between two sets of observations ($x1...n$ and $y1...n$). Correlations are simple, intuitive measurements that can be plotted on the x–y graphs we are first familiarized with at school. However, they describe average relationships (between groups) rather than individual relationships. They are therefore prone to confounding and cannot discern cause and effect.

A parametric correlation coefficient (Pearson's 'r') can be calculated if the data are near normally distributed and the relationship between the groups is approximately linear. Pearson's 'r' can be plotted on the x–y graph as a straight line, the gradient of which represents the correlation value (which is always between -1 and 1). This **Pearson correlation coefficient** is calculated as:

$$r = \frac{\sum(x - \bar{x})(y - \bar{y})}{\sqrt{\sum(x - \bar{x})^2 \sum(y - \bar{y})^2}}$$

Statistical significance is determined by calculating a t value as follows:

$$t = r\sqrt{\frac{n - 2}{1 - r^2}}$$

which has $n - 2$ degrees of freedom, and looking up a t table.

If either of the variables is not normally distributed, a **Spearman's rank** correlation coefficient is more appropriate. This is performed on the ranks of the observations (see Swinscow 1996 for the formula) and the significance is calculated as above.

Possible confounding of the correlation between normally distributed variables can be explored with **partial correlation** coefficients, but these can only control for the effect of a single potentially confounding variable per analysis.

If there is a linear relationship between two variables, then one can be designated the 'dependent variable' (y) and can be calculated from the other (the 'independent variable', x) by **regression**, using the regression equation:

$$y = a + bx$$

where **b** is the **regression coefficient** (calculated as above, without the $\sum(y - \bar{y})^2$ term in the denominator) and **a** is the **intercept** on the y axis. **a** is a constant which can be calculated as ($\bar{y} - b\bar{x}$). Note that any one value can be predicted from another, but that the linear assumptions may not apply beyond the data one actually has (e.g. age and height are linear in children but not in adults). Simple regression only looks at the effect of one independent variable, but the regression equation can be extended to include others in 'multiple regression', which is one of the most common multivariate techniques.

MULTIVARIATE STATISTICS

Multiple regression is the most common type of multivariate analysis as it can be employed when the dependent variable is continuous. As in any multivariate analysis, a measure of association is calculated taking a number of potential confounders into account simultaneously (e.g. age, sex, duration of illness, treatment, etc). In multiple regression this is done by simply extending the regression equation above:

$$y = a + b_1x_1 + b_2x_2 ....$$

provided that all the interrelationships between variables are linear (or can be rendered linear, by, for example, log or square transformations). The adequacy of a linear fit can be tested with a number of statistical techniques (see SPSS manuals). The coefficients in the model are calculated by 'least squares', where a regression line is fitted by minimizing the sum of the squared deviations between all the data points and the line.

If the dependent variable is binary (dichotomous), **logistic regression** is the technique of choice. Thus, the risk of developing an outcome (or not) is expressed as a function of independent predictor variables. The dependent variable is defined as the natural log of the odds of disease. If y is the probability of the disease, then $y/1 - y$ is the odds and the log odds is log $(y/1 - y)$ such that:

$$\log \frac{y}{1-y} = a + b_1x_1 + b_2x_2 + ...$$

These coefficients can readily be converted (as an antilog) into an odds ratio that is adjusted for confounding. The coefficients can also be converted into 'product terms' to assess interactions between independent variables, as would be required, for example, if age and sex exerted different combined effects in, say, young men and middle-aged women.

Other multivariate statistical tests merit at least a brief mention. Analysis of variance has a number of multivariate extensions: analysis of covariance, multivariate analysis of variance, and multivariate analysis of covariance. **Analysis of covariance** (ANCOVA) is essentially the same as multiple regression. **Multivariate analysis of variance** (MANOVA) is appropriate if one has a number of dependent variables of which to examine the associates, and **multivariate analysis of covariance** (MANCOVA) extends this when one wishes to examine the associations between multiple independent and dependent variables. MANOVA and MANCOVA are used to see if there are any statistically significant associations in the data set as a whole, before trying to identify them, as a method of avoiding multiple hypothesis testing. It is good practice to conduct and report a stratified analysis in subgroups of subjects (by ANOVA or the χ^2 test) before any multivariate procedures, to help identify and understand the confounders and their interactions. As a rough rule of thumb, for appraisal purposes, any multivariate technique is unlikely to be reliable unless there are at least 10 subjects for every variable entered into the analysis.

An alternative approach to examining large data sets is to use one of the types of **factor analysis** (e.g. principal components analysis) to identify groups of variables ('factors') that are highly intercorrelated and thus seem to be measuring the same underlying phenomenon, prior to conducting simpler analyses of the associations of the individual factors. Such 'data reduction' is, however, sensitive to interpretation, and one should always be careful in conducting and interpreting the analyses of such 'derived statistics'. Similar tests and principles can be applied to identify commonalities in groups of subjects (for example in 'latent trait analysis' and 'cluster analysis'), or to identify groups of variables and their interactions that determine the group status of subjects (e.g. in 'discriminant function analysis' and 'path analysis'). For example, factor analysis has identified three or more factors of schizophrenic symptomatology, cluster analysis has been employed to try to subtype depressive illness, and path analysis has been used to determine the various causes of the onset of depression.

This is a very brief account of a number of complex statistical techniques, each of which is the subject of many books. Interested readers can consult some fairly accessible resources for further details (e.g. Hennekens & Buring 1987, Duffy et al 1998, SPSS manuals), but should only attempt such analyses with experienced assistance.

SURVIVAL ANALYSIS

Survival analysis is a technique that merits special consideration as it is applied specifically to data from longitudinal cohort studies, in which one is interested in the time interval until an outcome occurs. The term was coined to give information on time to death in fatal conditions, but can be applied to any outcome (e.g. time to relapse). Commonly used statistics are the 'median survival rate', which is the length of time that 50% of the population with a particular disease will survive (or take to reach some other outcome), and the 1- or 5-year survival rates, which are the proportions of subjects still alive at those times. Such data are commonly presented as a 'life table'. They can also be plotted as a 'survival curve', which plots time on the x-axis and the proportion surviving (without the outcome) at each time point on the y-axis – and therefore has a stepped rather than a curved appearance (see Laupacis et al 1994 for examples). The cumulative proportion surviving at each time – $S(t)$ – is calculated by multiplying each proportion at each time point:

$$S(t) = \frac{r_1 - d_1}{r_1} \times \frac{r_2 - d_2}{r_2} \times \ ....$$

where r is the number alive (or without the outcome) and d the number dead (or with the outcome). This can also be expressed as $(1 - d_1/r_1) \times (1 - d_2/r_2) \ ....$

A key feature of this **Kaplan–Meier method** is that not all subjects reach the outcome at each data collection point, in which case the survival times are 'censored'. In other words, as $d = 0$ the product and the cumulative proportion are unaltered. This approach can be used to compare the survival of two populations who may or may not differ according to how they were treated etc. in a **log rank test**. As the times to outcome are unlikely to be normally distributed, this involves first ranking the data and then comparing the observed and expected outcome rates in each group, analogous to the χ^2 test (see Swinscow 1996 for details).

The log rank test cannot be used to explore or adjust for the effects of other variables. The multivariate extension is **(Cox's) proportional hazards regression analysis**. This is a type of logistic regression in which the independent variables are related to the log incidence rate of the outcome by including a time factor $a(t)$:

$$\log [\text{incidence rate } (t)] = a(t) + b_1 x_1 + b_2 x_2 + \ ....$$

The log incidence rate is generally referred to as the **hazard function**, which can also be expressed as the probability (hazard or risk) that an individual will experience an event in a time interval, allowing for prognostic variables.

As with any regression analysis the statistical output will present regression coefficients (b) which, if statistically significant, represent an increase or decrease in the chances of the outcome.

META-ANALYSIS STATISTICS

A meta-analysis simply calculates a summary effect size (usually OR or d) by taking the mean of all the individual study effect sizes 'weighted' by each study size to produce a weighted mean odds ratio or a weighted mean difference. Cochrane reviewers employ particular ('RevMan') software, which uses Peto's OR (a non-log transformed approximation to the OR, calculated as the difference between the observed and expected events divided by the variance) as this is best suited to meta-analyses on small studies. The rationale for weighting is that larger studies tend to be the most reliable estimates of any effect, as they sample more of the population. Weighting is done according to the standard error – the weight (Wi) of a study is simply the reciprocal of the standard error squared ($1/SE^2$).

The exact calculation of a mean effect size ($\bar{Y}$) can be done in various ways, but depends on whether one uses a fixed or a random effects model. **Fixed effects modelling** assumes that each study is an estimate of a single underlying effect (which therefore particularly favours large studies), whereas **random effects modelling** assumes that all included studies are a true random sample of all studies. Random effects modelling is generally preferable, as the assumption that there is no heterogeneity between studies in fixed effects modelling is not always safe. Indeed, if the P value of the heterogeneity ('Q statistic') test is less than 0.5 one is obliged to quote random effects, as the heterogeneity test is of low power (see below). Generally, however, the results from both models are reported and the smallest overall effect is regarded as most likely to be true (which is usually the random effects result).

Fixed effects calculation can be done according to the formula:

$$\bar{Y} = \frac{\sum \{ \frac{1}{SE^2}(\text{effect size})\}}{\sum \frac{1}{SE^2}}$$

Random effects calculation can be done according to the formula:

$$\bar{Y} = \frac{\sum (\frac{1}{SE^2} + \text{effect size}) \times (\text{effect size})}{\sum (\frac{1}{SE^2} + \text{effect size})}$$

The 95%CI of the mean weighted OR/d (Y) is: $Y \pm 1.96 \times SE$.

It should be obvious that including the effect size variance in the denominator in random effects modelling will generally reduce the summary estimate, as the effect size variance is by definition larger than the standard error.

Heterogeneity is a systematic difference in effects between studies beyond that expected by chance. If there is substantial heterogeneity between studies this can bias the summary effect, may reflect important methodological differences, and/or mean there are distinct subgroups of patients. It is therefore important to identify heterogeneity. This can be done by 'eyeballing' funnel plots or, quantitatively, by calculating the Q statistic in a heterogeneity test or by constructing a Galbraith plot.

Funnel plots are simple graphs of effect size (on the x-axis) against the precision of the estimate (SE or 1/SE), or just the number of patients (on the y-axis) – see Figure 3.2 for an example. Funnel plots were devised to evaluate the possibility of publication bias, but can also evaluate potential sources of heterogeneity. The rationale is as follows. Small studies (say $n < 30$) provide less accurate measures of effect than do larger studies, as they sample less of a population and are more prone to most types of bias. Therefore, small studies provide a wider scatter of results, whereas larger studies have greater precision and provide more similar measures of effect that are nearer to the true effect. If study size or standard error is plotted against effect size, the small studies will (in the absence of publication bias) be scattered along the bottom and the larger studies will aggregate at the top, giving a so-called (inverted) funnel shape. Plotting study size as 1/SE (precision) will give a funnel the right way up. In the presence of publication bias (i.e. small positive studies are published but not small negative studies) there will be an asymmetry of the funnel brim owing to an absence of small negative results (see Lawrie & Abukmeil 1998 for an example).

Funnel plots can also evaluate heterogeneity. If different types of study are given different symbols and the different symbols aggregate together, there is likely to be heterogeneity (see Geddes & Lawrie 1995 for an example).

The Q statistic is calculated as the weighted sum of all the differences between individual study effects and the overall effect, squared:

$$Q = \Sigma 1/SE_2 \times (\text{effect size} - \overline{Y})^2$$

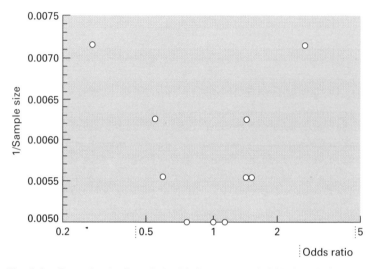

Fig. 3.2 **Example of a funnel plot** (circles represent individual studies).

which has the n of studies minus one degrees of freedom and a chi-square distribution.

A **Galbraith plot** can identify which studies contribute most to any overall heterogeneity. It is usually plotted as the z statistic (y-axis) against $1/SE$ (x-axis), such that larger studies (with small SE and larger $1/SE$) aggregate away from the origin. By representing different types of study with particular symbols, the source(s) of heterogeneity can be identified. Quantitatively, such studies will lie a certain number of standard deviations (usually 2) above or below the line that represents the summary effect (see Hotopf et al 1997 for an example).

Egger et al (1997) have suggested a method for quantifying any asymmetry and generating a P value for publication bias. They adapted the Galbraith plot by plotting the standard normal deviate (SND = OR/SE) against the precision ($1/SE$), with a regression line where SND = a + b × precision. In the absence of publication bias small studies will be close to zero on both axes (as SE will be large and both the SND and precision will therefore be low), whereas large studies will run with the true effect, i.e. $a = 0$ and b = the size and direction of effect. If there is publication bias the regression line will not run through the origin and the intercept provides a measure of asymmetry, with its 90%CI giving a P value (less than or greater than 0.1). The 90%CI and $P<0.1$ are chosen because these tests have low power, as they are generally comparing two groups of small numbers of studies. (Others have suggested simply performing rank correlations between the size of effects and their variances, but this is even less powerful.)

An additional way of quantifying the effects of publication bias is to calculate a 'failsafe n' of the number of negative 'desk-drawer' studies that would need to exist to render any significant overall effect non-significant.

COMMON STATISTICAL ERRORS IN PUBLISHED RESEARCH

Errors in the application of statistical tests or their interpretation are common in papers submitted for publication and in published studies. It has been recently estimated that about a half of all the papers which are approved by the peer reviewers of even prestigious medical journals such as the *Lancet* are seriously flawed in design, analysis or interpretation. A survey of published articles in the *British Journal of Psychiatry* came to the conclusion that about a half of the articles misused statistical testing (McGuigan 1995). In some cases this was simply using the wrong test for a particular type of data, which can have surprisingly little effect on the results (as so many of the tests are interrelated) but can be so seriously flawed as to cast doubt on the conclusions. Other common errors included multiple hypothesis testing and interpreting correlations as causal.

Multiple hypothesis testing can arise if there are multiple groups, multiple outcomes, repeated measures, subgroup analyses or interim analyses of the data. One can only be sure that this has not occurred in large data sets if plausible hypotheses are clearly stated, i.e. comparisons are planned at the design stage of the research and are therefore 'a priori'. If there are more than two groups, planned comparisons between the pairs of groups can be made 'a posteriori' in post hoc or follow-up tests. This is not the same as 'data dredging' for any significant differences, but it can be difficult to differentiate the two in practice.

Four further common sources of misinterpretation deserve particular mention: order effects, ceiling and floor effects, and regression to the mean. An 'order effect' (a systematic difference between first and subsequent assessments) occurs when one test is consistently given before another test, such that any differences between the tests may simply reflect the order in which they were done owing to any number of other factors (e.g. time of the day or month, fatigue, practice). 'Ceiling and floor effects' occur when a test result is so high or so low respectively (e.g. at the extremes of a scale with a restricted range), that it is very unlikely to be able to identify differences between two groups. 'Regression to the mean' is a similar, if more abstract concept. Stated simply, if any measure is repeated outliers are likely to tend towards the sample mean owing to measurement error.

The message if therefore clear: one cannot assume that the authors of published articles employ or interpret statistics correctly, and evaluating research requires appraisal of the statistics. This chapter, which may need to be read twice or more, should have given you the means to do this, but it is worth restating some general principles. The general rules of statistical testing and inference are: employ an appropriate test for the type and distribution of the data; use two-tailed significance testing; avoid multiple hypothesis testing or correct for it; always quote confidence intervals as well as P values; always consider the possibility of type I and/or II errors; and always consider possible biases and confounding.

RESOURCES

SPSS is the most commonly used statistical package in medicine, but there are several others commercially available (see Duffy et al 1998 for examples). There are also a number of useful programs that can be downloaded over the Internet, some of which are free. Arcus QuickStat (http://www.camcode.com/arcus.htm) is a general package which is particularly helpful for 'back of an envelope' meta-analysis, and can be used once as a free trial. It is just one of the facilities offered by StatsDirect (http://www.camcode.com). Epi Info is a series of programs for word processing, data storage and analysis that are freely available from the Center for Diseases Control in Atlanta (http://www.cdc.gov/epo/epi/epiinfo.com). G*Power is another free package which is designed to facilitate power calculations (http://www.psychologie.uni-trier.de:8000/projects/gpower/html). All of these sites also offer reasonably easy to follow information on the use of the packages.

REFERENCES AND FURTHER READING

Bland JM, Altman DG 1986 Statistical methods for assessing agreement between two methods of clinical measurement. Lancet i: 307–310

Duffy JC, Morrison DP, Peck DF 1998 Research design, measurement and statistics. In: Johnstone EC, Freeman CPL, Zealley AK (eds) Companion to psychiatric studies. Churchill Livingstone, Edinburgh, 149–196

Egger M, Davey Smith G, Schneider M, Minder CE 1997 Bias in meta-analysis detected by a simple graphical test. British Medical Journal 315: 629–634

Gardner MJ, Altman DG 1989 Statistics with confidence. BMJ Books, London

Geddes JR, Lawrie SM 1995 Obstetric complications and schizophrenia: a meta-analysis. British Journal of Psychiatry 167: 786–790

Gore SM, Altman DG 1982 Statistics in practice. BMJ Books, London

Hennekens CH, Buring JE 1987 Epidemiology in medicine. Little Brown & Co., Boston

Hotopf M, Hardy R, Lewis G 1997 Discontinuation rates of SSRIs and tricyclic antidepressants: a meta-analysis and investigation of heterogeneity. British Journal of Psychiatry 171: 87–91

Laupacis A, Wells G, Richardson WS, Tugwell P for the Evidence-Based Medicine Working Group 1994 Users' guides to the medical literature. V. How to use an article about prognosis. Journal of the American Medical Association 272: 234–237

Lawrie SM, Abukmeil SS 1998 Brain abnormality in schizophrenia: a systematic and quantitative review of the volumetric MRI literature. British Journal of Psychiatry 172: 110–120

McGuigan SM 1995 The use of statistics in the *British Journal of Psychiatry*. British Journal of Psychiatry 167: 683–688

Pocock, SJ 1983 Clinical trials: a practical approach. John Wiley & Sons, Chichester

Sackett DL, Haynes RB, Guyatt GH, Tugwell P 1991 Clinical epidemiology: a basic science for clinical medicine. Little, Brown & Co., Boston

Sackett DL, Straus SE, Richardson WS, Rosenberg W, Haynes RB 2000 Evidence-based medicine: how to practise and teach EBM, 2nd edition. Churchill Livingstone, London

Swinscow TDV 1996 Statistics at square one, 9th ed. BMJ Publishing, London

See also SPSS manuals and the series of occasional Statistics Notes in the *BMJ*.

REVISION MCQs

Q1 The following data require non-parametric statistics:

(a) Binary or dichotomous data

(b) Measures on an interval scale
(c) Measures on a ratio scale
(d) Data with a Gaussian distribution
(e) Measures on a nominal scale

Q2 The standard deviation:

(a) Is a measure of the distribution of data
(b) Equals the variance squared
(c) Is the denominator in the calculation of parametric effect sizes
(d) Is the same as the standard error in the general population
(e) Is equal to the standard error multiplied by the square root of the sample size

Q3 The following are parametric statistical tests:

(a) The t test
(b) Analysis of variance
(c) The χ^2 test
(d) Multiple linear regression
(e) Proportional hazards regression

Q4 A power calculation may use the following:

(a) Data from previous studies
(b) An α value of 0.8
(c) A β value of 0.8
(d) An estimate of the effect size
(e) An estimate of the numbers in the study

Q5 Odds ratios:

(a) Compare outcomes in exposed and non-exposed populations
(b) Are calculated from a contingency table as ad/bc
(c) Are the same as relative risks
(d) Of 1.0 mean that there is no difference between groups
(e) Range from minus to plus infinity

Q6 The following statements about confidence limits are true:

(a) They are a measure of precision

(b) The 95% confidence interval is calculated as the effect plus and minus 1.96 times the standard error
(c) They give the same information as the P value
(d) The wider they are the better
(e) The confidence interval of an odds ratio involves logarithms

Q7 The following statements about regression are true:

(a) The regression equation ($y = a + bx$) can be used to calculate the value of a dependent variable from that of an independent variable
(b) Multiple regression is applicable if the relationships between variables are linear
(c) Logistic regression is applied to dichotomous outcome variables
(d) Cox's proportional hazards regression is a multivariate test
(e) Multiple regression can evaluate the role of confounders

Q8 The following methods can be used to evaluate the possibility of publication bias in a meta-analysis:

(a) A funnel plot
(b) Calculating the number of unpublished positive findings
(c) The Q statistic
(d) The confidence interval of the summary effect
(e) A Galbraith plot

ANSWERS

A1

(a) True
(b) False
(c) False
(d) False
(e) True

A2

(a) True
(b) False (it is the square root of the variance)

(c) True
(d) False
(e) True (as SE = SD/$\sqrt{n}$)

A3

(a) True
(b) True
(c) False
(d) True
(e) False

A4

(a) True
(b) False (α is usually 0.05 or lower)
(c) False (β is usually 0.2 or lower, as $1 - \beta$ equals the power)
(d) True
(e) False (a power calculation generates rather than uses the estimated numbers)

A5

(a) True
(b) True
(c) False (they are calculated differently)
(d) True
(e) False (they range from zero to infinity)

A6

(a) True
(b) True
(c) False (they also give information on precision)
(d) False (narrow limits mean greater precision)
(e) True

A7

(a) True
(b) True
(c) True

(d) True
(e) True

A8

(a) True
(b) False (the number of negative findings is relevant)
(c) False (this is a test for heterogeneity)
(d) False (this measures the precision of the estimate)
(e) True (although it requires adaptation)

4

Critical appraisal

Critical appraisal requires some knowledge of research methods and statistics but is equally dependent upon common sense. It is possible to rote-learn the checklists of useful questions to ask for each type of study that one might encounter, but far preferable to apply a few basic principles sensibly. The first task is to decide what sort of study is being evaluated, although it is usually obvious whether diagnosis or treatment etc. is being considered. One must then decide whether a given paper is scientifically valid, i.e. is the design suitable for the issue being addressed; are the research methods sufficiently rigorous; and are any statistical tests appropriate? If it is valid, one can then use some of the concepts and numbers devised by evidence-based practitioners to determine whether any findings are clinically important and applicable.

This chapter describes the appraisal of the most common types of study of relevance to psychiatrists. We do so in the order that one might deal with a particular clinical problem, i.e. starting with diagnosis and ending with guidelines and audit. We have used clinically relevant examples throughout, starting with a likely clinical scenario and appraising a relevant paper, to facilitate understanding. We provide checklists of useful questions to ask about each type of study, adapted from those of Sackett et al (2000), as a guide to appraisal rather than something to be forced into your memory. They should not therefore be rote-learned, and in some instances differ from the questions asked in the text.

As you read this chapter you may find it useful to read the paper(s) appraised in each section, but we have reproduced the essential details here (as far as copyright laws allow) and the chapter is therefore self-contained. Finally, we should reiterate that what is written here is very likely to be far more than you are required to know to pass the exam, as it is also designed as a reference source for the rest of your professional life. Do not, therefore, despair if you find the following more conceptually alien and mathematically complex than you envisaged. Be prepared to read things through more than once, and try to understand the text rather than memorize it.

DIAGNOSIS

As with most studies, the critical appraisal of articles on diagnosis can be facilitated by answering three major questions (Roman et al 1994a, b). The first asks 'Is the study valid?', and is a necessary prerequisite before considering the article any further. The second question is 'Is the study important?', and is answered by looking at the reliability and performance of the diagnostic test using clinically relevant measures. The third and last question is 'Can I use this study in caring for my patient(s)?', and is the final step before applying the results of a diagnostic study in your clinical practice. We will now go through diagnosis following these three major headings.

Clinical scenario

You are called to the emergency department of a psychiatric hospital one night to see a man who is acting 'strangely'. You are asked to assess him to ascertain whether or not he suffers from a mental illness. You notice he is wearing numerous layers of clothing and you recall a recent paper (Arnold et al 1993) suggesting that this may be indicative of schizophrenia. You set about finding this article after you have seen the patient, who seems to be suffering from a psychotic illness manifested by third-person auditory hallucinations and progressive self-neglect.

Précis of published article

The study was conducted at a psychiatric emergency room in Memphis. All patients referred there were assessed by an unstructured interview, and subsequently staff were asked to record whether patients were wearing redundant clothing. All staff remained blind to the hypothesis. The study was conducted for 9 months, ending when 25 redundantly clothed patients had been obtained. There were 549 non-redundantly clothed people with schizophrenia and related diagnoses identified, as well as 1471 non-schizophrenic persons also without redundant clothes. Of the total 25 patients who wore redundant clothing, 18 received a diagnosis of schizophrenia and seven did not. This is in contrast to 2020 non-redundantly clothed controls, 549 (27%) of whom received a diagnosis of schizophrenia and 1471 (73%) who did not. The authors stated that, although not particularly sensitive, redundant clothing is a readily observable behaviour associated with schizophrenia in the emergency room.

Is the study valid?

Question 1 Has there been a blind comparison with a gold standard?

When deciding whether data about a diagnostic test are useful or not, it is important that the test has been compared against a gold standard, the results of which can be relied on to give a true account of whether or not the diagnosis is present. Psychiatry is sometimes criticized for having few gold standards, as the majority of diagnoses are based on information from the history and mental state examination. However, structured clinical interviews, generating diagnoses based on operational criteria, are frequently used as gold standards when evaluating a diagnostic test. In order for this to be done reliably without the person applying the diagnostic test or gold standard being influenced by the findings of the other test, the comparison must be ' blind'.

The paper does not address this point, and the diagnostic test seems to have been compared with the gold standard in an open fashion by the same individual administering the unstructured interview. Although the paper states that clinicians were blind to the study's hypothesis, blind comparison with a 'gold standard' structured clinical interview would have been a much more rigorous methodological approach. The bias introduced by non-blinding is likely to overestimate the value of the diagnostic test.

Question 2 Was the test evaluated in an appropriate group of patients?

When assessing whether data about a diagnostic test might be useful to you as a clinician or purchaser, it is important that the data were obtained on patients like those in whom it would be used in practice. Data derived from patients in the late stage of an illness, e.g. chronic schizophrenia, where the diagnosis may be relatively obvious, may not be particularly informative. Ideally the diagnostic test should have been applied to a range of patients with early and late disease, mild to profound in severity, and of different ages, some of whom were receiving treatment whereas others were treatment free. It is also an advantage to have the test applied to patients with diagnoses frequently confused with the target disorder. For example, in a study examining the use of a diagnostic test for schizophrenia it would be an advantage also to have applied the test to people with bipolar disorder, as this is a common differential diagnosis.

The paper is evaluated in an emergency room of a North American hospital. You surmise that this may be different from an emergency department in a UK psychiatric hospital, but it seems similar enough for the data to apply.

Question 3   Was the gold standard applied regardless of the test result?

Sometimes when a positive test has been obtained from a diagnostic test, investigators are tempted not to proceed with the gold standard. This is especially the case where the gold standard is particularly risky, expensive or labour intensive. The reverse may also occur, whereby patients who have been found to have a particular result on the gold standard do not have the diagnostic test applied. This may result in vital information being omitted about the diagnostic test and will seriously bias some of the measures used to assess its importance.

The study in question seemed to apply the gold standard test irrespective of the diagnostic test in question until 25 people with redundant clothing had been recorded.

Is the test important?

When deciding whether or not a diagnostic test is useful in your own clinical practice, the consequences of a positive and a negative test in the study need to have been thoroughly examined. A patient who has a negative test result but who has the target disorder (a false negative) is an important omission and may lead to important treatment being withheld. Similarly, a patient without the target disorder but who has a positive test (a false positive) may be subject to needless anxiety, further investigation and unnecessary treatment. Objective measures of a test's performance can be obtained by placing the data from a diagnostic test in a contingency (2×2) table as follows:

Table 4.1   A 2 × 2 table of redundant clothing as a diagnostic test for schizophrenia

| Diagnostic test | Gold Standard Schizophrenic disorder | | |
	Yes	No	Total
Redundant clothing			
Positive	18 (a)	7 (b)	25 (a + b)
Negative	549 (c)	1471 (d)	2020 (c + d)
Total	567 (a + c)	1478 (b + d)	Total = a + b + c + d

Question 1   What is the sensitivity of the test?

The people who have the disorder and who have a positive test are called true positives. The proportion of people with the disorder who have a positive test is called the sensitivity of the test and this is assumed to be a constant property of the test. A sensitive test is one in which a positive result identifies most people with the target disorder. Hence, when a sensitive test is used a negative test tends to rule out the disorder (SNout).

Algebraically,

Sensitivity = Proportion of people with the illness $(a + c)$ who have a positive result (a).

$$\text{Sensitivity} = \frac{a}{a+c}$$

In this case the total number of people with the disorder is 567 and the proportion of those with a positive test is 18. Therefore the sensitivity is 18/567, which is 0.032 (3.2%).

Question 2   What is the specificity of the test?

The people who do not have the disorder and who have a negative test are called true negatives. The proportion of people without the disorder who have a negative test is called the specificity of a test, and is assumed to be constant. A specific test is one in which a negative result identifies most people without the disorder. Hence, when a specific test is used a positive test tends to rule in the disorder (SPin).

Algebraically,

Specificity = Proportion of people without illness $(b + d)$ who have a negative test (d).

$$\text{Specificity} = \frac{d}{b + d}$$

In this case the total number of people without the disorder is 1478 and the proportion of those with a negative test is 1471. Therefore the specificity is 1471/1478, which is 0.995 (99.5%).

Question 3   What is the positive predictive value?

In clinical practice, when a diagnostic test is positive it is useful to know what proportion of subjects will truly have the disorder. The proportion of people with a positive test who have the disorder is called the positive predictive value (PPV). This is not a constant property of a test, as it rises as the total prevalence of disorder increases.

Algebraically,

PPV = Proportion of people with a positive test $(a + b)$ who have the illness (a).

$$\text{PPV} = \frac{a}{a + b}$$

In this case the total number of people with a positive test is 25 and the proportion of those with the disorder is 18. Therefore the positive predictive value is 18/25, which is 0.72 (72%).

Question 4   What is the negative predictive value?

When a diagnostic test is negative it is useful clinically to know what proportion of those with a negative test will truly be free of the disorder. This is called the negative predictive value (NPV). It is not a constant property of a test, as it rises as the total prevalence of disorder decreases.

Algebraically,

NPV = Proportion of people with a negative test $(c + d)$ who *do not* have the illness (d).

$$\text{NPV} = \frac{d}{c + d}$$

In this case the total number of people with a negative test is 2020 and the proportion of those without the disorder is 1471. Therefore the negative predictive value is 1471/2020, which is 0.728 (72.8%).

Question 5   What is the likelihood ratio for a positive test?

The likelihood ratio of a positive test result is useful in determining its clinical utility, as it can be used like the PPV/NPV to indicate the value of a given test result but is calculated from the sensitivity and specificity, so that it is generally constant for a given testing location. The likelihood ratio for a test result is **the value that result has in predicting the presence of the disorder**. Therefore, the likelihood ratio (LR) of a positive test result is the value of a positive test in increasing the suspicion that an individual has the disorder, and is usually >1.

Algebraically,

$$LR+ = \frac{\text{Prob (positive test from someone with the disorder)}}{\text{Prob (positive test from someone without the disorder)}}$$

$$LR+ = \frac{a/(a+c)}{b/(b+d)}$$

$$LR+ = \frac{sensitivity}{1-specificity}$$

In this case the sensitivity is 18/567 and (1–specificity) is 7/1478. Therefore, the LR+ is 18/567 multiplied by 1478/7. This figure is 6.7.

Question 6   What is the likelihood ratio for a negative test?

Similarly, the likelihood ratio of a negative test result is the probability of a negative test in those with the disorder divided by the probability of a negative test in those without the disorder, and is usually less than 1 if the test is useful in excluding the disorder. A likelihood value of less than 1 means that a negative test result is more likely to come from someone without the disorder than someone with it. Theoretically, a likelihood ratio of 0 would mean a negative result would have no value in predicting the presence of disorder, but would be perfect in predicting its absence.

Algebraically,

$$LR- = \frac{\text{Prob (negative test from someone with the disorder)}}{\text{Prob (negative test from someone without the disorder)}}$$

$$LR- = \frac{c/(a+c)}{d/(b+d)}$$

$$LR- = \frac{1-sensitivity}{specificity}$$

In this case (1–sensitivity) is 549/567 and specificity is 1471/1478. Therefore, the LR– is 549/567 multiplied by 1478/1471. This figure is 0.97, and therefore very close to unity.

Note on diagnostic thresholds

Although not always a consideration in diagnostic studies, it is convenient to mention at this point the issues that determine where a diagnostic threshold should be set, as they relate closely to the other mathematical and clinical measures mentioned so far. When a measurement is used to make a diagnosis, whether of a biological parameter or of a reading on a rating scale, the decision as to which rating or measurement should signify a positive diagnostic result is not straightforward. Higher cut-offs generate more specific but less sensitive tests, and lower cut-offs more sensitive tests that are less specific. When deciding which diagnostic threshold to choose, clinical circumstances are an essential consideration, as are whether the cost of false negatives or false positives is the greatest. The costs of false negatives are greatest when patients have a poor prognosis if untreated but where there is a safe, inexpensive and effective therapy. In these circumstances a highly sensitive test is warranted. The costs of false positives are greatest where patients with a positive result are subjected to further unpleasant, expensive investigations and treatment offers limited benefit. In cases where the costs of false positives and false negatives have equal consequences, the receiver operator characteristic (ROC) curve may be particularly useful (Figure 4.1). The curve is constructed by plotting the sensitivity against 1–specificity for each diagnostic cut-off. In these circumstances it is possible to capitalize on both sensitivity and specificity so that their average ([sensitivity + specificity]/2) is at its maximum value. This maximum value is attained at the cut-off nearest to the shoulder (or 'knee') of the ROC curve.

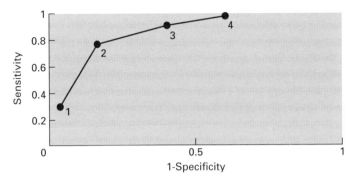

Fig. 4.1 **A receiver operator characteristic curve.**

The ROC curve can also be used to compare competing diagnostic tests. The overall performance of a test is reflected by the area under the curve. Superior tests generally have a greater area under the curve. Similarly, the likelihood ratios for a positive and a negative test can be used to compare different diagnostic tests.

Can I use the diagnostic test in caring for my patients?

Having decided whether the study is valid and whether the results are important, you then need to decide whether it can be used clinically. There are a number of issues to address.

Question 1 Is the diagnostic test available, accurate, affordable and precise in your setting?

The availability of a test is obviously an important prerequisite for its implementation. Even if a diagnostic test is available in your setting, the expertise necessary for its performance may not be. Similarly, a diagnostic test may perform accurately among psychiatrists in a psychiatric centre, but is not necessarily as accurate when used by other professionals in primary care; the reverse may equally be the case. Expensive tests may be justified when the test correctly identifies people with a disease that is common, serious and treatable; however, in other circumstances the financial cost may outweigh the benefits. Finally, as we discussed when considering validity, a test studied in patients with severe and chronic illnesses may not be applicable to your own clinical population in which the test is to be used (i.e. first-episode cases). The likelihood ratio for a positive test will tend to be greater for a population that contains severe and enduring disorders than for one in which new admissions are being assessed for the first time. It may be possible to make sensible estimates of the sensitivity and specificity in your population to examine whether the test will be useful in clinical practice. This type of exploration is known as a sensitivity analysis (see below).

The test 'redundant clothing' would obviously be widely available in any situation. It is affordable and there seems no reason to suppose that it will be any more inaccurate than in the situation in which it was first used. However, the main value of the test lay in ruling the disorder in when redundant clothing was present. It missed the vast majority of people with the disorder and would almost certainly be of extremely limited usefulness as a single diagnostic test (although this does not of course mean that the test has no clinical value whatsoever).

Question 2   Can you generate a clinically reasonable estimate of your patients pretest probability?

If the study in which the test was first evaluated has a prevalence of the disorder similar to your own the test can be expected to behave similarly. However, if the test will be used in a patient population where the prevalence of the disorder is less than that in the study (e.g. primary rather than secondary care), the value of a positive test will be less likely to indicate the presence of the disorder (i.e. the post-test probability will fall). A useful way of calculating how a test will behave in your clinical setting is to use likelihood ratios. First, you will need to estimate the prevalence of the disorder in your population, preferably by studying your practice population or by reviewing the psychiatric literature. If data are not available from these sources, personal speculation may be an alternative but less satisfactory option.

Algebraically,

Because

$$\text{Odds} = \frac{P}{1-P} \quad \text{then} \quad P = \frac{\text{Odds}}{1+\text{Odds}}$$

In the above paper there are 567 people with schizophrenia and 1478 without – 2045 in total. The prevalence of schizophrenia is therefore 567/2045, or 0.28 (28%). From the above equation the pretest odds are 0.28/(1 − 0.28), or 0.39. However, if only 10% of those presenting to your service for emergency assessment have schizophrenia, the pretest probability, or prevalence, is therefore 10% or 0.1, and the pretest odds are 0.1/(1−0.1) or 0.11.

Therefore, for any pretest probability (i.e. the prevalence of the target disorder in your sample) the pretest odds can be calculated. From these and the likelihood ratio calculated earlier, we can calculate the post-test odds. From this we can calculate the post-test probability, which is the prevalence of the disorder in those who have a positive test. **The post-test probability is a useful estimate of the positive predictive value in your own patients**.

Algebraically,

$$\text{Post-test odds} = \text{likelihood ratio} \times \text{pretest odds}$$

Therefore, given any prevalence and LR, post-test odds and probability can be calculated.

Example
If the prevalence of schizophrenia in our sample were 10%, what would be the post-test probability of (a) positive and (b) negative test results ?

(a) Post-test probability of a positive result

We have calculated the LR+ = 6.7.
The prevalence in our sample is 10%, therefore:

$$\text{Odds} = \frac{P}{1-P} = 0.1/0.9 = 0.11$$

Post-test odds   = pretest odds × LR+
                    = 0.11 × 6.7 = 0.74

And, as

$$P = \frac{\text{Odds}}{1+\text{Odds}}$$

Post-test probability = 0.74/(1 + 0.74) = 0.43 (43%).

This means that in your own patients 43% of those with a positive test will have the disorder.

(b) Post-test probability of a negative result

We have calculated the LR– = 0.97.
The prevalence in our sample is 10%, therefore:

$$\text{Odds} = \frac{P}{1-P} = 0.1/0.9 = 0.11$$

Post-test odds
$$= \text{pretest odds} \times \text{LR–}$$
$$= 0.11 \times 0.97 = 0.11$$

And, as

$$P = \frac{\text{Odds}}{1+\text{Odds}}$$

Post-test probability = 0.11/(1 + 0.11) = 0.099 (9.9%).

This means that in your own patients, 9.9% of those with a negative test will have the disorder (false negatives). Put another way, this means that 90.1% of those with a negative test will not be schizophrenic (true negatives). The post-test probability for a negative test is an estimate of 1–negative predictive value (1–NPV) in your own patients. However, as 90% of people are free from the illness anyway, the negative test result does not take us much further forward. Indeed, diagnostic tests are rarely very useful if the prevalence of the disorder in a given clinical situation is <10% or >90%.

These calculations are rather involved and post-test probabilities can be calculated from a nomogram (see Figure 4.2). This is used to calculate post-test probabilities by first anchoring a point on the pretest probability line and another on the likelihood ratio. The post-test probability is then calculated by reading off the value on the right-hand axis.

If several tests are applied in sequence to a patient, the post-test odds can be estimated by multiplying the pretest odds by all of the likelihood ratios for the tests used. Therefore, if a patient had a positive result on three separate tests, called A, B and C, the likelihood ratio for all three positive tests could be calculated thus:

Combined likelihood ratio for a positive result =
$(\text{LR}_A+) \times (\text{LR}_B+) \times (\text{LR}_C+)$

Question 3   Will the the test affect your management and help
your patient?

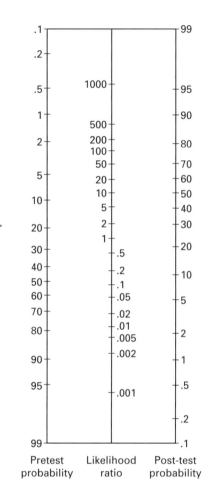

Fig. 4.2 Diagnosis nomogram for Bayes' theorem.

The performance of the test in your own situation and the consequences of having the disorder will be crucial in deciding whether the test will affect your management. If the test generates very large post-test probabilities it will have ruled in the disorder. The patient may then have crossed a test–treatment threshold where effective management of that disorder can begin. However, low post-test probabilities may lead to further diagnostic tests until a treatment threshold is reached.

Likelihood ratios are very useful for this purpose, as individual LRs can be multiplied with each other to produce a composite LR. Sometimes a test with a relatively low likelihood ratio may be justified. The use of the CAGE alcohol-screening question-naire with a positive diagnosis set at one affirmative answer may be one such example. The use of the questionnaire at this level may lead to many people without alcohol problems being positive for the test, but few people with the disorder will be missed. The test may be justifiable: first, because patients with alcohol problems have an identified effective treatment (simple advice to reduce consumption); secondly, the costs of missing the disorder are high; thirdly, because the test is so simple and can be performed by almost everyone, the cost involved in terms of money and time is low. Finally, but most importantly, it is vital that the diagnostic test must be acceptable to patients. In summary, the costs of diagnosis both to the patient in terms of physical pain and stigma, and to society in terms of resource allocation, must be balanced against the benefits to the patient and society at large.

The test in the study we have appraised has very low sensitivity but 99.5% specificity. It may be useful in ruling in the disorder when the redundant clothing 'sign' is present. However, in your own clinical practice, if only 10% of referrals have schizophrenia only 43% of those with a positive test will have the target disorder, and 90.1% of those without redundant clothing will not have the disorder.

Conclusions

You decide that although the study has methodological weaknesses it is probably valid. Having found that it has high specificity and low sensitivity you decided to see how it would perform in your own patients. You found that approximately 57% of people with a positive test would not have schizophrenia. In those who do not have a positive test some diagnoses (9.9%) would be missed if this were the only means of investigation in a sample where the prevalence of schizophrenia was 10%. Therefore, a full clinical examination would still have to be conducted. You note that the presence of redundant clothing should increase your suspicion that someone may be suffering from schizophrenia, but that it has minimal clinical utility.

Diagnosis worksheet

Is the study valid?

1. Was there an independent, blind comparison with a reference ('gold') standard of diagnosis?
2. Was the diagnostic test evaluated in an appropriate spectrum of patients (like those in whom it would be used in practice)?
3. Was the reference standard applied regardless of the diagnostic test result?

Is the study important?

		Target disorder		Totals
		Present	Absent	
Diagnostic test result	Positive	a	b	a + b
	Negative	c	d	c + d
	Totals	a + c	b + d	a + b + c + d

Sensitivity = $a/(a + c)$ =
Specificity = $d/(b + d)$ =

Likelihood ratio for a positive test result = LR+ = $sens/(1-spec)$ =
Likelihood ratio for a negative test result = LR– = $(1-sens)/spec$ =

Positive predictive value = $a/(a + b)$ =
Negative predictive value = $d/(c + d)$ =

Pretest probability (prevalence) = $(a + c)/(a + b + c + d)$ =
Pretest-odds = $prevalence/(1-prevalence)$ =

Post-test odds = pretest odds × likelihood ratio
Post-test probability = post-test odds/(post-test odds + 1)

Can I use the study in caring for my patient(s)?

Is the diagnostic test available, affordable, accurate and precise in your setting?

Can you generate a clinically sensible estimate of your patient's pretest probability (from practice data, from personal experience, from the report itself, or from clinical speculation)?

Will the resulting post-test probabilities affect your management and help your patient? (Could it move you across a test–treatment threshold? Would your patient be a willing partner in carrying it out?)

Would the consequences of the test help your patient?

TREATMENT

The critical appraisal of a single treatment study follows the same three major questions (Guyatt et al 1993, 1994). The first asks 'Is the study valid?', and is a necessary prerequisite before considering the article any further. The second question is 'Is the study important?', and is answered by looking at the size of the treatment effect using clinically relevant measures. The third and last question is 'Can I use this study in caring for my patient?', and is the final step before applying the results of a treatment study in your clinical practice.

Clinical scenario

A long-stay patient with chronic schizophrenia continues to complain of persistent and disabling auditory hallucinations despite an adequate trial of clozapine. Having heard that cognitive behaviour therapy (CBT) may be effective in the treatment of chronic schizophrenia, you wonder whether your patient might benefit from it. You review the literature and find a randomized controlled trial of CBT versus supportive psychotherapy (Tarrier et al 1998) and you set about critical appraisal of this article.

Précis of published article

Chronic schizophrenic patients were randomly allocated, stratified according to sex and severity of symptoms, to intensive CBT and routine care, supportive counselling and routine care, or routine care alone. Positive symptoms were assessed at baseline and 3 months after treatment using the brief psychiatric rating scale (BPRS). The number of patients showing a 50% improvement in symptoms (BPRS score) was the main outcome measure. Assessors were blind to which treatment was being received and the randomization list was kept in sealed envelopes throughout the study. Patients were analysed according to the groups to which they were randomized, and the supportive psychotherapy and CBT groups were matched for therapist time. Eighty-seven patients entered the study, 72 completed treatment, and a further seven were able to provide complete data. For the remaining eight, their last observed ratings were carried forward. Of 33 patients in the CBT 11 showed a clinically significant improvement, compared with four out of 26 in the supportive psychotherapy group and three of 28 in the routine care group. This difference was significant when patients who showed 50% or more improvement were compared with those who received CBT and the other two groups combined.

Is the study valid?

Question 1 Were the patients randomized to the treatments, and was the randomization list concealed?

The reasons for randomization are to reduce bias and to ensure that confounders are distributed randomly between the two groups. Of course, chance confounding may occur where a factor associated with a particular outcome is unevenly distributed; however, the probability that this will happen is no greater than chance. Studies using non-random allocation tend to introduce bias and overestimate treatment effects. It is also important that the randomization process is adequate: allocating alternate patients to treatment or control is an inadequate method and can lead to bias being introduced. Having adequately randomized patients to treatment or control, it is highly desirable that the list is concealed from those carrying out the trial. Experimenters may consciously or unconsciously introduce bias if they are aware of the groups to which patients have been randomized.

Having examined your study, it appears that patients were randomized adequately at the beginning using a 'stratified block randomized procedure' (this means that patients were randomized in blocks according to a particular characteristic, to ensure that this would be balanced across the three treatment groups). It is also stated in the text that the randomization list was concealed from patients and clinicians in sealed envelopes by a third party.

Question 2   Were the groups similar at the start of the trial?

Differences in confounding variables can occur in the groups at the beginning of a trial that may affect the response to treatment. For example sex, length and severity of illness, previous treatment and comorbid substance misuse may all affect response to antipsychotic medication in schizophrenia. It is important, therefore, that differences between groups are minimal at the outset of a trial. If the groups have been adequately randomized, differences in confounding variables will not usually be significant, although chance differences may occur.

The study shows a table of two possible confounding variables, the number and severity of symptoms. Patients were stratified according to symptom severity. Chance differences could have occurred between the groups as a result of the randomization procedure, such as social background differences, but this is not stated. An important possible confounder was medication, but the authors say that 'there was no evidence of systematic and significant differences between the groups in terms of medication'.

Question 3   Were the groups treated equally apart for the
             treatment in question?

The purpose of a clinical trial is to examine the effect of an intervention. If groups are treated unequally in some other regard it is impossible to exclude the possibility that this may be an important part of any differences in outcome. For example, for patients in a drug trial it is important that both groups are otherwise dealt with by the researchers with equal enthusiasm. Otherwise, the effect of social interaction itself may cause one of the groups to have a greater response to the treatment. Equal treatment in clinical trials is particularly difficult when psychotherapy is the intervention being used. Patients in the placebo group must receive equal amounts of therapist time and receive an intervention that seems to be plausible. Patients who believe they belong to the placebo group are (generally) less likely to respond and more likely to leave the study prematurely.

It appears that in this study therapist time was controlled for and that the active and supportive psychotherapy control groups were treated equally. Supportive psychotherapy and CBT may have been different between patients, but an attempt was made to ensure the fidelity of treatment, i.e. the treatments were given as they should be (see primary article for further details).

Question 4   Were clinicians and patients 'blind' to which intervention was being received?

Clinicians may introduce bias to a trial if they are aware of the treatment group to which a patient belongs. They may do this either consciously or unconsciously. They may treat the active group differently from the control group, or they may interpret the results of the treatments in accordance with their expectations. Either way, they may seriously prejudice the validity of a study.

The current study states that clinicians and investigators were blind to the active treatments. Asking raters to guess which group a patient belonged to tested this possibility. Apparently they were able to do this no better than by chance alone. Patients in the 'treatment as usual' group were more likely to have assumed they were in the inactive limb of the study. The supportive psychotherapy group was matched for therapist time and received treatment according to a preset protocol. It is therefore unlikely that these patients were aware that they belonged to a control group, although the authors could have tested this by asking patients to guess whether they were receiving the active or the control treatments.

Question 5   Were all the subjects who entered the trial accounted for at its conclusion?

Ideally, all patients who enter a trial complete it. This is rarely the case, however, as patients may be lost from both groups for a variety of reasons, including protocol violation, side effects, or even following a dramatic response to therapy. Deciding how many patients can drop out of a study before the results are jeopardized is difficult. The journal *Evidence-Based Mental Health* insists on 80% follow-up (end-point assessment), but the most important consideration in how to interpret dropouts is the use of intention-to-treat analysis. This analyses people in the groups to which they were originally randomized, whether they completed the trial or not. Thus, individuals who drop out of the study are usually regarded as treatment failures, to minimize the chances of dropouts biasing the overall results. If treatment dropouts were excluded from the analysis then the results would tend to overestimate the effect of treatment.

Sometimes when a dropout occurs a study will use a last observation carried forward. This assumes that the last measurement, for example on a symptom rating scale, provides an accurate estimate of what that person's rating would have been at the end of treatment. However, a treatment response is frequently followed by a subsequent return to the original or baseline value on a scale, such that the last observation carried forward may be an unduly optimistic estimate. For this reason the classification of dropouts as treatment failures is based upon safer (more conservative) assumptions than the last observation carried forward.

The study in question seems to account for all the patients at the beginning and end of the trial. An intention-to-treat analysis was made and the last observation was carried forward for seven subjects who could not provide complete data. You have misgivings about this, but do not feel that it invalidates the study.

Is the study important?

When deciding whether a study is clinically important, the use of some simple mathematical concepts is useful. In order to make this process easier some people use a simple contingency (2×2) table to highlight the figures needed for calculation. These can be used when an outcome is dichotomous, e.g. remission vs. non-remission, and when there are two or more treatment groups. If the rows always represent treatment groups and the columns always represent outcomes, mistakes are less easily made (Table 4.2).

Question 1   What are the control event rate (CER) and the experimental event rate (EER)?

Studies may measure outcome in a number of ways. The first, and arguably the least clinically useful, is using a continuous measure such as a symptom rating scale. These studies can produce

Table 4.2 Comparison of patients experiencing improvement in psychotic symptoms on CBT versus supportive psychotherapy

| | Outcome | | |
Treatment	Improvement	Non-improvement	Total
CBT	11(a)	22(b)	33
Controls (SP)	4(c)	22(d)	26
Total	15	44	59

important effects, and a useful statistic called the **effect size** can be calculated. The second and probably most clinically useful method is to measure a clinically relevant dichotomous outcome such as admission or readmission, dead or alive, relapse or non-relapsed. In these cases it is possible to obtain a figure called the **control event rate** (although it can be more usefully thought of as a ratio). This is simply the frequency of the event in question in the control group, and is calculated by dividing the number of control subjects experiencing an event by the total number of control subjects. In our example the rate of improvement in the control group is 4 out of 26 (15.4%, or 0.15). This figure is the control event rate (CER). The **experimental event rate** is similarly the event rate in the treatment or active group, and is calculated by dividing the number of experimental subjects experiencing an event by the total number of experimental subjects. In our example 11 out of 33 subjects improve in the experimental (CBT) group. Therefore the EER is 11/33 (33.3%, or 0.33).

Question 2 What are the absolute benefit increase (ABI), relative risk (RR) and relative benefit increase (RBI)?

In studies that examine a favourable event it is possible to calculate a figure called the **absolute benefit increase**. This is done by subtracting the rate of desirable events in the control group from that in the experimental group.

Algebraically,

Absolute benefit increase = experimental event rate – control event rate

$$ABI = EER{-}CER$$

In studies in which an effective treatment is compared on a negative outcome, for example relapse, the control event rate will generally be larger than the experimental event rate. For this reason the term **absolute risk reduction** (ARR) is used instead, and is calculated from the difference between experimental and control event rates.

In our example the event in question is improvement; the CER = 0.15 and EER = 0.33. Therefore, ABI = 0.18 or 18%. This means that there is an 18% increase in the rate of improvement attributable to the effect of treatment.

The **relative risk** – a familiar concept to those acquainted with epidemiology – is simply the risk of the event in question in the active or experimental group divided by the risk of the same event in controls.

Algebraically,

$$\text{Relative risk} = \text{EER/CER}$$

$$\text{RR} = \text{EER/CER}$$

The **relative benefit increase** statistic expresses the absolute increase in benefit attributed to the treatment as a proportion of the risk in controls. It is calculated by dividing the absolute benefit increase by the control risk (CER), or by subtracting 1 from the relative risk.

Algebraically,

$$\text{Relative benefit increase} = \frac{\text{Absolute benefit increase}}{\text{Risk in controls}}$$

$$\text{RBI} = \frac{\text{EER} - \text{CER}}{\text{CER}}$$

Or,

$$\text{RBI} = \text{RR} - 1$$

Therefore, in our example the relative benefit increase is (0.33–0.15) or 0.18, divided by 0.15, which is 1.2. This means that experimental subjects are 1.2 times more likely to improve than are control subjects.

Question 3 What is the number needed to treat?

The **number needed to treat** (NNT) is a very important statistic designed to measure the efficacy of a treatment in a clinically relevant and intuitive way. It is calculated from the reciprocal of the absolute benefit increase (ABI) or absolute risk reduction (ARR), and is a statement of how many people need to be given the active treatment in this study to prevent one event that would have occurred had they been treated with the comparison treatment.

Algebraically,

Number needed to treat = Reciprocal of the absolute benefit increase

$$\text{NNT} = 1/\text{ABI}$$

In our example the absolute benefit increase was calculated to be 0.18, therefore the number needed to treat is 1 divided by 0.18, which equals 5.6 or 6. An NNT is usually quoted as a whole number and rounded up, as it refers to numbers of patients. An NNT of 6, in this example, means that six people need to be treated with CBT to bring about one extra improvement compared with supportive psychotherapy.

Generally, an NNT of <10 is regarded as clinically significant. However, if a particularly severe outcome is prevented, or where a treatment is applied to very large numbers of people (such as a public health measure), NNTs much greater than this may also be clinically important. In studies where the outcome of interest is time to an event, calculations can be extended to show the number needed to treat at any time point after the start of treatment (Altman & Anderson 1999).

Confidence intervals on the absolute risk reduction and number needed to treat. Having calculated the ARR and NNT, it is possible to measure the precision of these estimates using confidence intervals. The 95% confidence limits are usually quoted, and these represent the interval within which we can be 95% certain that the true value lies. If the confidence interval for an ARR crosses 0, or that for an NNT crosses infinity, the results may be attributable to chance alone. With all confidence intervals their values are based upon the standard error of the parameter.

The standard error of an ARR is:

$$\sqrt{\frac{\text{CER}(1-\text{CER})}{n_1} + \frac{\text{EER}(1-\text{EER})}{n_2}}$$

(n_1 = number of control subjects, n_2 = number of experimental subjects.)

The 95% confidence interval is the ABI ± 1.96 × standard error (ABI$_{min}$ to ABI$_{max}$). The 95% confidence limits on an NNT are simply the reciprocals of these two ARR confidence limits.

In this example:

$$SE = \sqrt{\frac{0.15 \times 0.85}{26} + \frac{0.33 \times 0.67}{33}} = 0.11$$

95%CI for the ARR = ABI ± 1.96 × SE = 0.18 ± 0.22, or −0.04 to 0.4.

The 95%CI for the NNT is 1/ARR$_{max}$ to 1/ARR$_{min}$ or −1/0.04 to 1/0.4, or approximately −25 to 2.5.

This shows that the ARR and NNT are not statistically significant and have a wide confidence interval. The authors get around this problem by combining the two control groups in order to obtain a statistically significant result. Otherwise, the results of the study could be attributed to chance alone.

Question 4   What is the odds ratio for improvement on the active treatment?

Odds ratios are frequently quoted in studies as a measure of treatment effect size. Their use is not particularly intuitive, but odds ratios from several studies can be combined to form a more precise estimate of efficacy, in the case of meta-analysis. Odds ratios can also be used to calculate the NNT in your patients if the event rate in your untreated individuals is known. This measure is known as the **patient expected event rate** (PEER) and is a substitute for the CER (see next section).

The odds ratio is the ratio of the odds that patients will improve on active therapy other than the control treatment. The odds of an event is the probability that an event will occur divided by the probability that it will not occur.

Algebraically,

$$Odds = \frac{Probability\ that\ an\ event\ will\ occur}{Probability\ that\ an\ event\ will\ not\ occur}$$

Or,

$$Odds = \frac{P}{1-P}$$

The odds ratio is therefore:

$$\text{Odds ratio} = \frac{\text{Odds of improvement on active treatment}}{\text{Odds of improvement on control treatment}}$$

$$\text{OR} = \frac{\text{Odds (improve/active)}}{\text{Odds (improve/control)}}$$

In our example we can see that the odds of improvement with the control treatment are the rate of improvement using the control treatment (CER) divided by 1 minus this figure (1–CER). This is 0.15/0.85, or 0.18. We could have calculated this figure from our table as (*a*) divided by (*c*). The odds of improvement on the active treatment are similarly the rate of improvement with active treatment (EER) divided by 1 minus this figure (1–EER). This is 0.33/0.67 or 0.49, and could have been calculated from our table as (*b*) divided by (*d*). The odds ratio is therefore the odds of improvement on treatment divided by the odds of improvement on the control therapy. This figure is 2.7; this means a patient treated with CBT is 2.7 times more likely to improve **than not**, compared with patients treated with supportive psychotherapy. We could have calculated it from our table thus:

Algebraically,

$$\text{Odds ratio} = \frac{\text{Odds of improvement on active treatment}}{\text{Odds of improvement on control treatment}}$$

Odds of improvement on active treatment $= a/b$
$\qquad\qquad\qquad\qquad\qquad$ [or EER/(1–EER)]
Odds of improvement on control treatment $= c/d$
$\qquad\qquad\qquad\qquad\qquad$ [or CER/(1–CER)]

Therefore,

$$\text{OR} = \frac{a/b}{c/d}$$

And

$$\text{OR} = \frac{ad}{bc}$$

In this example,

$$\text{OR} = ad/bc = (11 \times 22)/(4 \times 22) = 2.7$$

Confidence interval for an odds ratio. The precision of an odds ratio estimate can also be measured using a confidence interval, in much the same way as it is used to calculate the confidence interval for an ABI or NNT.

The standard error for the natural log of an odds ratio is:

$$\sqrt{\frac{1}{a} + \frac{1}{b} + \frac{1}{c} + \frac{1}{d}}$$

The 95% confidence interval for an odds ratio is therefore the antilog of the natural log of the odds ratio minus 1.96 times the natural log of the standard error to the odds ratio plus 1.96 times the natural log of the standard error. This can be calculated from the data given in Table 4.2.

Can I use this study in caring for my patients?

Having decided a study is both valid and important, it is necessary to decide whether you can apply it to your particular patient. To do this it is useful to ask the following questions.

Question 1 Do these results apply to my patient?

The patient in your ward or clinic is unlikely to have been included in a clinical trial that answers your question. Therefore, you will have to assess whether the patients in the trial are sufficiently like your own to provide useful information. If your own patient would have been *excluded* from the trial in question because of their age, illness, comorbidity or other clinical reason, applying the results to them will require extrapolation. Judging whether the results still apply to your patient is a matter of clinical experience and factual knowledge.

Question 2 How great would the potential benefit be for my patient?

Having identified a useful, valid and important study that appears to apply to your patient, how can you estimate the likely benefit they will derive from this treatment? If your patient is taken from a sample similar to that used in the trial, and appears to be as susceptible to the outcome in question as those stated in the trial, the results may also apply to your patient. This is often not the case, but one can use the results of the trial to estimate what the NNT will be for patients like yours in one of three ways.

Method 1
The first step in estimating the NNT for your patients is to estimate the **patient expected event rate** (PEER). This is the susceptibility or baseline risk patients like yours have for the outcome in the study. If, for example, the study examined relapse rates in schizophrenia over a 1-year period on chlorpromazine rather than to placebo, you would need to estimate how susceptible your patients are to relapse over a 6-month period on placebo. This can be estimated from clinical experience, from studies of prognosis or (arguably best of all) from your own locally collected audit data. Having calculated this figure and expressed it as a fraction or percentage, you can multiply it by the **relative benefit increase** (RBI) to give a new absolute benefit increase. The RBI is derived from the primary study and is assumed to be constant, and the new ABI can be used to calculate the NNT for your patients by taking the reciprocal.

Worked example 1
You wish to know what the likely benefit is from CBT in your patients. The benefit you wish to give your patients is improvement. Having found a suitable study you estimate from local data that the rate – or risk – of improvement in your patients receiving stable treatment (but no CBT) over a 1-year period is 5%. What is the NNT of CBT for your patients?

$$PEER = 0.05 \qquad\qquad RBI = 1.2$$
$$ABI_{new} = RBI \times PEER = 0.05 \times 1.2 = 0.06$$
$$NNT_{new} = 1/0.06 = 16.6 \text{ (17 to the nearest figure)}$$

Therefore, 17 of your patients need to be treated to produce one improvement in your sample.

Method 2
The simpler but less accurate method to use when calculating NNTs for your patients starts with an estimation of the relative susceptibility to an outcome in those not exposed to the treatment. The resulting relative susceptibility is expressed using the letter F (for 'fraction') in the following way.

For example, $F = 2$ would mean that your patients are twice as susceptible to the outcome as those in the trial, whereas $F = 0.5$ would mean your patients are half as susceptible to the outcome as those in the trial. The NNT for your patient is simply the NNT reported in the trial divided by the value of F.

Worked example 2

Using the data in worked Example 1, you estimate that your patients are half as likely to improve as those in the trial (based on the fact that your patients are also resistant to clozapine treatment). What is the NNT for your patients?

$$F \quad = \quad 0.5$$
$$NNT_{old} = \quad 5$$
$$NNT_{new} = \quad 5/0.5 \qquad \text{Therefore, } NNT_{new} = 10$$

Therefore, 10 of your patients will need to be treated with CBT to prevent one relapse. You decide to use Method 1 however, and accept the figure $NNT = 17$.

Method 3
Alternatively, a nomogram can be used to avoid the use of a calculator (Figure 4.3).

Question 2   Is the treatment compatible with your patient's values and preferences?

Having decided the treatment is valid, important, and can potentially produce a sizeable clinical effect, the next step is to decide whether it is compatible with your patient's values and preferences. Painful treatments for inoperable cancer may have small NNTs to prevent death in 1 month, but this difference may not be compatible with your patient's goals, which might be more influenced by the relief of pain. Similarly, some patients may not consent to ECT for depression, even if relevant high-quality trial information is available.

There are many other considerations when deciding whether a treatment should be used or not. Side effects play a major role and are covered in the next section. Economic analyses may also be important when deciding whether the cost of a treatment justifies its use, when less expensive and equally effective alternatives exist elsewhere. Economic analysis is also covered in a subsequent section.

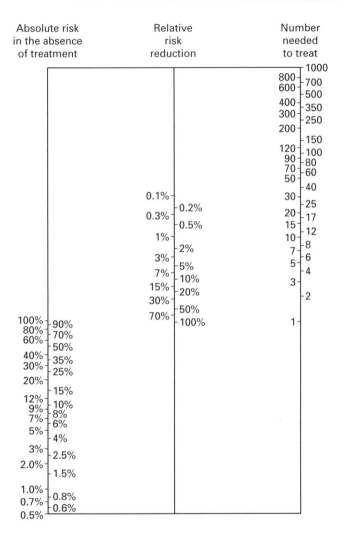

Fig. 4.3 Treatment nomogram for Bayes' theorem.

You decide, however, that CBT is compatible with your patient's preferences and goals and arrange for the treatment to be carried out on an outpatient basis.

Conclusions

CBT for chronic treatment-resistant schizophrenia appears to have been validly studied in a double-blind, randomized controlled trial.

It also produces important results which, you estimate, are likely to be experienced by patients in your own clinical practice. It seems that they would be prepared to undergo the procedure. Although a meta-analysis would be a greater recommendation still, you decide to adopt CBT for treatment-resistant schizophrenia, and eagerly await the results of studies that examine the economic and any harmful consequences of this treatment.

Further steps in evidence-based treatment

There are two further steps in evidence-based practice that are not, strictly speaking, part of critical appraisal. First, the evidence must be implemented, and secondly there should be an ongoing process of evaluation and audit. These processes are essential if our efforts at critical appraisal are to be worthwhile. Furthermore, to ensure that our knowledge does not become out of date, and that are treatments are quality controlled, there must be a continual process by which we evaluate our clinical practice.

Therapy worksheet

Is this study valid?

Was the assignment of patients to treatments randomized? Was the randomization list concealed?

Were all patients who entered the trial accounted for at its conclusion? Were they analysed in the groups to which they were randomized?

Were patients and clinicians kept 'blind' as to which treatment was being received?

Apart from the experimental treatment, were the groups treated equally?

Were the groups similar at the start of the trial?

Is this study important?

Occurrence of outcome		Relative risk reduction (RRR)	Absolute risk reduction (ARR)	Number needed to treat (NNT)
Control event rate (CER)	Experimental event rate (EER)	$\dfrac{\text{CER} - \text{EER}}{\text{CER}}$	CER − EER	1/ARR

95% confidence interval (CI) on an NNT = 1/(limits on the CI of its ARR)

$$\text{Standard error of an ARR} = \sqrt{\dfrac{\text{CER} \times (1 - \text{CER})}{n_1} + \dfrac{\text{EER} \times (1 - \text{EER})}{n_2}}$$

(n_1 = number of control subjects, n_2 = number of experimental subjects.)

Therefore, the 95%CI for ARR is:

ARR (best estimate) $\pm$ 1.96 × standard error (ARR_{max} to ARR_{min})

The 95%CI for an NNT is $1/\text{ARR}_{max}$ to $1/\text{ARR}_{min}$.

Can I use this study in caring for my patients?

Do these results apply to your patient?	
Is your patient so different from those in the trial that its results can't help you?	
How great would the potential benefit of therapy actually be for your individual patient?	
Method 1: F	Risk of the outcome in your patient, relative to patients in the trial.
	Expressed as a decimal: _____
	NNT/F = _____/_____ = _____
	(NNT for patients like yours)
Method 2: 1/(PEER × RRR)	Your patient's expected event rate if they received the control treatment:
	PEER:_____
	1/(PEER × RRR) = 1/_____ = (NNT for patients like yours)

Can I use this treatment in caring for my patient(s)?

Do you and your patient have a clear assessment of their values and preferences?	
Are they met by this regimen and its consequences?	

HARM

Harm refers to the adverse effects of an agent. Commonly encountered harmful exposures in psychiatry include aetiological factors and therapeutic treatments. Several types of study can be used to assess the harmful effects of an exposure (Levine et al

1994), the main studies being randomized controlled trials, cohort and case–control studies, and case series. These can also be used to study the impact of potential aetiological factors, with the exception of randomized controlled trials, as this would be unethical.

A randomized controlled trial is, at least theoretically, the study of choice for assessing the harmful effects of an agent, in much the same way as it is used to assess the therapeutic potential of others. There may be practical and ethical problems with such a design. For example, it would be unethical to randomly allocate a patient to something one suspects to be harmful, such as randomizing subjects to 'smoking' or 'non-smoking' groups to assess damage caused by tobacco. Practical problems also arise when the harmful event is not very common. A large number of subjects will be required to detect a few who will develop the particular adverse event. If a drug caused depression in 1% of people where the prevalance of depression in the population is 5%, the number of patients required to show this effect would be very large.

A cohort study of harm or aetiology involves prospectively comparing those individuals exposed to a possibly harmful agent with those unexposed. The two groups are then followed to monitor the incidence of the adverse event of interest between the groups. This is ethically acceptable, as an intentional exposure was not created, and is useful for uncommon exposures as the people who are exposed and not exposed already exist, and may be selected in large numbers. However, there may be differences between the two groups at the outset of the study, which should be taken into account. For example, if the suicide rate were compared in patients attending a general adult psychiatrist with those who do not, the risk would appear greater in those receiving psychiatric treatment. However, such a study would be confounded by the presence of a psychiatric illness. Statistical correction for confounding variables may be possible, but there may be other prognostic differences between the groups which cannot be corrected for, especially where important risk factors are unknown. Finally, where a study aims to examine a rare outcome, the numbers of subjects needed for a cohort study may be very large. For this reason a case–control study may be more practical.

In case–control studies 'cases' with the outcome of interest are identified. This could be disease or death. Researchers then choose a group of control subjects who do not have the outcome of interest but who are otherwise similar to the cases. The cases and controls are followed back, retrospectively, to look for exposure to harmful agents which could explain the affliction. However stringently the controls may be collected, there may still be important differences in confounder levels between the groups. The researchers know the outcome and are therefore not blind. They may be biased towards identifying a harmful exposure among the cases more than controls, and subjects may be more prone to recall exposures more carefully when an adverse outcome has already occurred. One great advantage of this design, however, is that it can be used to detect relatively rare events or outcomes that may take years to manifest. This is because unaffected individuals do not have to be studied until the event occurs, as the cases are selected from those with the outcome of interest already in the population.

Case series and reports may be the first published accounts of aetiology or harm, and may lead on to more systematic investigations. Such studies are fraught with bias, as patients are non-randomized, and uncontrolled, and there is an obvious tendency for studies that show an effect to be written up and published more often than those that do not. However, such studies at the very least show that the outcome and exposure can occur together, even though a cause and effect relationship may not exist, and may be the only practical design for very rare events.

Clinical scenario

You have often heard it said that pregnant women should not take lithium because of the risk of cardiac anomaly in the fetus. Recently, you treated a female patient who relapsed after her lithium was discontinued during pregnancy. For future reference you wish to know the degree of risk to the fetus with lithium. You identify a cohort study (Jacobson et al 1992) from the literature and decide to appraise the article.

Précis of published cohort study

The researchers prospectively recruited and followed 148 women using lithium during the first trimester of pregnancy. Pregnancy outcome was compared with that of controls matched for maternal age. Complete follow-up was achieved in 138 out of 148 women. Rates of major developmental abnormalities did not differ between the lithium (2.8%) and the control (2.4%) groups. Birthweight was significantly higher in the lithium-exposed infants (P = 0.02). These results suggest that lithium is not an important human teratogen.

Is this study valid?

Question 1 Was the diagnosis of the disease well defined?

As with other study designs there should be inclusion and exclusion criteria for selecting the members of a cohort. In the case of a disease or disorder operational diagnostic criteria should be used wherever possible. The operational criteria will define the clinical features required for the diagnosis, and also increase diagnostic reliability. Exclusion criteria can be any clinical condition that could confound the results. Common confounders in psychiatry include physical illness and substance misuse.

In this study congenital cardiac malformations were diagnosed using fetal echocardiography and post-delivery echocardiography. No criteria for diagnosis are stated. It would have been useful to mention that the diagnoses were based on a protocol, if one was used.

Question 2 Was the source of the cases described?

A cohort should ideally be a representative group for the particular illness. Knowing the source of cases helps us to estimate how representative the cohort is compared with the cases one is likely to encounter in clinical practice. For instance, depression in primary care is different in its course and outcome from that which is treated in secondary and tertiary care. One good test of 'representativeness' would be to check whether the number of cases in the cohort is in keeping with the incidence figures of the particular condition in that population. If a condition has a documented incidence of 1% then a representative cohort from a catchment area of 5000 will not yield more than 50 new cases a year. However, not all the cases will enter a study, for various reasons such as underreporting or refusal to participate.

The cases in this study were 148 clients who were enrolled when they contacted a teratogen information service with concerns about lithium. This is not an ideal source. Ideally, all the pregnant women in a particular area would have been screened for lithium treatment. The sample in this study may therefore have been biased by factors determining whether a pregnant woman would consult such a service (e.g. social class, intelligence, past history, etc.).

Question 3 What efforts were made to ensure complete ascertainment of cases?

Apart from selecting cases from proper sources, thorough procedures should be adopted to ensure that all cases are contacted for the study. Missed cases reduce the similarity between the cohort and the real population of cases. This would limit the extrapolation of study findings to the target population, and may introduce bias.

The cases in this study were clients who were enrolled when they contacted one of the four teratogen information services. In essence, these were women who had been proactive in seeking information on teratogenic drugs and, by that virtue, perhaps more careful about drug intake in general (including alcohol and other drugs). However, the 148 controls were also recruited using the same technique as those concerned about other drugs without any known therapeutic potential.

Question 4 Were exposures and outcomes measured in the same way in the groups?

Both experimental and control groups need to go through the same processes of evaluation for the study to be valid. If the experimenters are not completely blind to the assignment of subjects to each group, there may be some tendency to measure exposures and outcomes more thoroughly in the group at risk. This would result in more frequent detection of cases in the exposed group. This can be prevented if it is clearly stated how exposure and outcome will be measured, and objective assessments are obviously preferable.

Both the cohorts in this paper were followed up after delivery in the same manner.

Question 5 Were there initial differences between the groups, and were these corrected?

Because a cohort study does not have random assignment to the experimental and control groups there may be intrinsic differences between the groups (e.g. age, or exposure to some other toxin). In this study, if the ages of the lithium-exposed mothers were higher it would put them at a higher risk for delivering babies with congenital malformation, and lithium might be falsely attributed as the cause. It is important to apply statistical corrections if such differences are found. In this study there is no difference in maternal age or medical/obstetric history between the groups. It may also be useful to identify any differences within each group. This would help to analyse outcomes in terms of subgroups for a clearer association between the risk and any subgroup character- istics.

Question 6   Was exposure measured in an objective manner?

The importance of this has already been mentioned. This is to ensure that little or no bias occurs in the reporting and collection of information from subjects. Information could also be collected from other sources, such as medical records and patients' GPs. Objective methods also help to ensure that assessments will be done in the same manner by all investigators. If possible, the degree of exposure should also be measured. For example, in a harm study involving cigarettes or alcohol, the quantity used would be important to record.

In this example information was collected from patient records and GPs, but there is no mention of serum lithium levels, although these may have been measured.

Question 7   Is there a temporal relationship between the cases and the exposure?

Where an event precedes an exposure, the exposure obviously cannot be causal. Similarly, when an exposure takes place 20 years before an event, the exposure is less likely to be causal than when the period between the exposure and event is considerably less. For this reason it is important to take into account the temporal relationship between the exposure and outcome when deciding whether the results of a study of harm are valid. Clearly some agents can exert a harmful effect many years later (e.g. maternal influenza exposure may increase the risk of schizophrenia), and the biological plausibility of the relationship needs also to be considered.

With respect to lithium's putative teratogenic effects, one should be able to pick up any obvious damage to the fetus at the time of delivery or soon after.

Question 8   Is there a dose–response gradient?

A dose–response gradient between an exposed agent and the severity of adverse effect greatly supports the aetiological link. It may also allow one to stratify risk based on the level of exposure. For example, there is a dose-dependent risk of liver damage with increasing alcohol intake. In this case it might have been informative to relate the lithium levels with the number or severity of congenital anomalies, but this was not done.

Is the study important?

Many studies quote results in the published text, without the use of tables. However, the use of a contingency (2×2) table may frequently be helpful, and one is included here (Table 4.3).

Table 4.3   Contingency (2×2) table of lithium and the risk of congenital abnormality

Exposure to lithium	Congenital abnormality	
	Present	Absent
Yes	4 (a)	134 (b)
No	3 (c)	145 (d)

Question 1   What is the relative risk?

Relative risk (RR) compares the incidence of adverse events in those exposed with that in those unexposed.

$$RR = \frac{\text{incidence among exposed}}{\text{incidence among not exposed}}$$

$$RR = \frac{a/a + b}{c/c + d}$$
$$= a(c + d)/c(a + b)$$
$$= 4 \times 148/3 \times 138$$
$$= 1.3$$

Note that *ad/bc* will give you approximately the same answer when *a* and *c* are small numbers, because adding *c* to *d* and *a* to *b* does not change the results much. We can therefore use this formula (*ad/bc*), (i.e. **the odds ratio**), for events with a relatively low incidence (this is called the **rare disease assumption**). This statistic is also used in case–control studies, where the incidence rates in the exposed and the unexposed are unknown.

In this study exposure to lithium confers 1.3 times the risk of malformation than no exposure.

Confidence intervals for the relative risk.   In order to calculate the precision of a relative risk estimate, one must calculate the confidence intervals. If such intervals are wide the estimate will be less precise than if they are narrow. Similarly, if the interval crosses zero the results are statistically insignificant and may be due to chance alone.

The formula for the calculation of a relative risk is based upon the calculation of the standard error ('unit of uncertainty'). The natural log of the standard error for a relative risk is given by:

$$\log_e SE = \sqrt{\frac{1}{a} + \frac{1}{b} - \frac{1}{n_1} - \frac{1}{n_2}}$$

(*a* and *b* are the numbers of people experiencing the event in the exposed and unexposed groups of size n_1 and n_2).

The confidence interval for a natural log of the relative risk is therefore the natural log of the relative risk (best estimate) ± 1.96 × natural log of the standard error. In this example, the standard error is:

$$\log_e SE = \sqrt{\frac{1}{4} + \frac{1}{3} - \frac{1}{138} - \frac{1}{148}} = 0.75$$

Therefore, the 95% confidence limits are:

$$\text{anti-log} [\log_e (1.3) + 1.96 \times 0.75 \text{ to } \log_e (1.3) - 1.96 \times 0.75] = 0.3 \text{ to } 5.6$$

As the confidence interval crosses 1 it is not statistically significant.

Question 2 What is the number needed to harm?

In studies where an agent significantly increases the risk of an adverse event, the number of patients needed to be exposed to bring about one additional adverse event can be calculated, as a clinically useful measure. This is called the number needed to harm (NNH), and is calculated by subtracting the risk of the adverse event in the control or non-exposed group from that in the experimental or exposed group. This figure is known as the absolute risk increase (ARI). The reciprocal of this figure is the NNH.

This does not apply to the current study as the risk was not significantly increased. However, the absolute risk increase is 4/138 – 3/148, or 0.0087. The reciprocal of this is 114.7 (115, to the nearest whole figure). Therefore the number needed to harm is 115.

Confidence intervals on the number needed to harm. In the same way that confidence intervals can be calculated for a number needed to treat, confidence intervals can also be calculated for the absolute risk increase and the number needed to harm. The interested reader may like to adapt the earlier equations for this purpose.

Can I use this study in caring for my patient(s)?

Having identified a valid study with important results, you must then decide whether its results apply to your patient(s). This decision can be made on the basis of the answers to four questions.

Question1 Can the results be extrapolated to my patient(s)?

The issue here is whether your patients are so different from those in the study that the results do not apply. Patients may not have met the inclusion criteria set in the study, but it is reasonable to suppose that the results may apply in some cases.

Our clinical scenario concerns a patient with a psychiatric illness who was currently taking lithium. She stopped because of the supposed risk to her fetus, but no adverse event occurred. She is unlike the subjects in the study in that she was not consulting a fetal screening service and there may be other differences in health behaviour that might affect her risk of fetal abnormality. However, she is not so unlike the patients in the study that the results do not apply.

Question 2 What are your patients' risks of the adverse outcome?

You may recall that we earlier calculated an NNT for your patient from the patient expected event rate (PEER) and the relative risk reduction. The situation for a cohort study is almost exactly the same. The relative risk increase may be calculated from the difference in event rates in the exposed and non-exposed cohorts, divided by the risk in the non-exposed. The PEER is the rate of the adverse event in unexposed patients, and is calculated from the published literature, clinical experience or clinical audit data. If the relative risk increase is calculated and the PEER is known, then the NNH for patients like yours can be calculated from the following formula.

Algebraically,

$$NNH_{new} = \frac{1}{RRI \times PEER}$$

The NNH can also be calculated using the F (fraction) statistic, which estimates how susceptible patients like yours are to the adverse outcome in question, in a similar way to a treatment study. Theoretically, a nomogram similar to that given in Figure 4.2 could also be used, though they are less often used in this context.

You decide to use the first method to estimate the NNH for patients of your own. Therefore, suppose the rate of fetal abnormality in patients like yours was 5%, compared with approximately 2% in the published article. The relative risk is 1.3; therefore, the relative risk increase is 0.3 (RRI = RR – 1). Then,

$$NNH_{new} = 1/(0.3 \times 0.05) = 66.7$$

Therefore, you would need to treat 67 patients with lithium to cause one additional adverse event that would not otherwise occur.

However, some cohort studies give an odds ratio rather than a relative risk increase. In this case a more complicated calculation must be used.

Algebraically,

$$NNH = \frac{[PEER \times (OR - 1)] + 1}{PEER \times (OR - 1) \times (1 - PEER)}$$

You decide that an NNH of 67, although large, for such a severe and distressing outcome should not be ignored. However, you also remember that the relative risk was not statistically significant and that the estimate was not very precise (from the 95% confidence limits). The relative risk may therefore be much less (or much greater) than the estimate you are using.

Question 3 What are your patients' preferences, concerns and expectations from this treatment?

Studies of harm must be interpreted in accordance with your patients' preferences and expectations. Where an exposure has no potential therapeutic benefit the decision may be to avoid exposure, where there are no other considerations. However, where an exposure has a therapeutic benefit the decision to continue with treatment or seek an alternative will depend on the degree of risk and the willingness of the individual to endure it. Patients may sometimes be risk-averse and accept little risk, or be prepared to accept massive risks because of the therapeutic benefit. A composite measure of the likelihood of being helped/harmed (LHH) can be helpful (see Sackett et al 2000 for further details).

You decide that an NNH of 67 may be acceptable to some pregnant mothers, but that the majority would probably be risk-averse when carrying a fetus in the first trimester of pregnancy.

Question 4 What alternative treatments are available?

In cases where the number needed to harm is clinically significant, it is important to identify what alternatives are available. This is especially the case if the number needed to treat exceeds the number needed to harm. Alternatives should include pharmaco-logical, non-pharmacological, and no interventions whatsoever. If a patient experiences a rare but specific adverse event to a drug (e.g. neutropenia with clozapine) it may be straightforward to change to another therapy. In other cases (e.g. sedation with antipsychotic medication) the potential risks and benefits of alternative medications may be more difficult to weight.

You understand that the main alternatives to lithium for bipolar disorder are anticonvulsants, antipsychotics, psychologically orientated treatments, and no treatment at all. You are aware of evidence of effectiveness for some of the above treatments. You are also aware that anticonvulsants are also possible teratogens. You decide that you will review the evidence for fetal anomaly with these treatments and present the evidence to future patients in an understandable format, so that they can make truly informed choices between therapeutic options.

Conclusion

Having reviewed this cohort study it appears that its conclusions are valid, potentially important, and may apply to your patients. Some doubt remains in your mind about the estimate of relative risk and you await a meta-analysis or larger cohort study in this important area.

Harm/aetiology worksheet

Are the results of this study valid?

1. Were there clearly defined groups of patients, similar in all important ways other than exposure to the treatment or other cause?

2. Were treatment exposures and clinical outcomes measured the same ways in both groups (e.g. was the assessment of outcomes either objective [e.g. death] or blinded to exposure)?

3. Was the follow-up of study patients complete and long enough?

4. Do the results satisfy some 'diagnostic tests for causation'?

   - Is it clear that the exposure preceded the onset of the outcome?

   - Is there a dose–response gradient?

   - Is there positive evidence from a 'dechallenge–rechallenge' study?

   - Is the association consistent from study to study?

   - Does the association make biological sense?

Are the results important?

		Adverse outcome		
		Present (case)	Absent (control)	Totals
Exposed to the treatment	Yes (cohort)	a	b	a + b
	No (cohort)	c	d	c + d
	Totals	a + c	b + d	a + b + c + d

In a randomized trial or cohort study

$$\text{relative risk} = RR = [a/(a+b)]/[c/(c+d)].$$

In a case–control study

$$\text{odds ratio (or relative odds)} = OR = ad/bc.$$

In this study:

Can I use this study in caring for my patient(s)?

---

1. Can the study results be extrapolated to your patient?

---

2. What are your patients' risks of the adverse outcome?
   To calculate the NNH for any odds ratio (OR) and your patients' expected event rate for this adverse event if they were NOT exposed to this treatment (PEER):

$$NNH = \frac{[PEER \times (OR-1)] + 1}{PEER \times (OR-1) \times (1-PEER)}$$

---

3. What are your patients' preferences, concerns and expectations from this treatment?

---

4. What alternative treatments are available?

PROGNOSIS

Prognosis is the outcome of a disease or a disorder and prognostic factors are relevant factors that influence the outcome. They can be demographic (e.g. age), disease specific (e.g. mood-incongruent delusions in depression) or comorbid conditions (e.g. depression with drug abuse). Prognostic factors are associated with the disease but do not necessarily cause the disease or disorder. Risk factors, on the other hand, are factors that predispose to or precipitate a disease (e.g. head injury and dementia) but do not necessarily act as maintaining or prognostic factors. Studies of prognosis may be appraised according to a series of questions (Laupacis et al 1994).

Typically, cohort studies and case–control studies are used to describe prognosis and to identify particular or putative prognostic factors. Rigorously performed randomized trials can also be used to study prognosis, but as most trials use criteria-based selection of patients, who may differ from the typical patient population, the results are likely to be less generalizable.

Clinical scenario

You are posted in a state hospital as a part of your psychiatric rotation. You notice that that there is a lot of discussion about the prediction of further criminality after discharge. There are no clear regional figures or data in the textbooks, but you identify the following article from a MEDLINE search: 'Criminal conviction after discharge from special hospital' (Buchanan 1998).

Précis of published article

A cohort of 425 patients discharged between 1982 and 1983 from a special hospital were selected. Criminal records of these patients were obtained for the next 10.5 years from the Offenders Index through the Research and Statistics Department of the Home Office: 24% had reoffended within 5.5 years, with 9% convicted of serious offences, 8% of violent offences and 5% of sexual offences; 31% had reoffended within 10.5 years, with 14% convicted of serious offences, 4% of violent offences and 7% of sexual offences. A legal category of psychopathic disorder was the most important predictor of reconviction. Prior criminal record had only a small effect on reconviction. Other factors, such as gender or destination of discharge, had no influence on reconviction.

Is this research valid?

Question 1   Is the sample representative and were the patients selected without bias?

To obtain a true idea about prognosis you would like the patients to be representative of the group in general. The use of diagnostic criteria and structured assessments improves the fidelity of psychiatric diagnoses. It is important to remember, however, that such extensive diagnostic examinations are not routinely carried out in clinics and may identify a narrow band of patients. You would also like to know whether the subjects are from a service similar to your own.

This paper includes the type of subjects you have in your setting. It does address your question, but people may offend without being convicted, such that reconviction is not the same as reoffending. The cohort includes all patients who were discharged in a given time frame, and should therefore be unbiased. Note, however, that the author does not use standard clinical diagnostic descriptions but legal categories such as psychopathic disorder and mental impairment. Note also that there is no control group. Released prison inmates without documented psychiatric illness would have been a good comparison group.

Question 2 Were the patients identified at a common point of their illness?

Although patients in a study may be similar to yours in terms of diagnosis, it is important to ascertain at which stage they are in the course of their illness. For example, patients with bipolar affective disorder have an increase in the frequency, duration and intensity of episodes later in the course of the illness. If the cohort is composed of patients with a longer duration of illness then the prognosis will generally be poorer than in a cohort earlier in the course of their illness. However, this may not be true of particular issues, including criminal behaviour, as this may be more strongly associated with first episodes of psychosis.

The patients in this cohort have different diagnoses and also appear to have a wide range of ages. They have all entered the hospital at different points of their illness. However, the author does report results specific to the age of the patients.

Question 3 Was the follow-up of patients sufficiently long?

Prognosis studies measure the rates of negative or positive events in the cohort. However, a particular event may not happen within the duration of the follow-up period, especially if it is short.

This study follows up the cohort for 10 years, which is a fairly long period. The results show a reasonable frequency of the event of interest (reconviction) during the follow-up period.

Question 4 Were objective criteria applied in a blind manner?

The outcomes of interest should be stated objectively at the beginning of the study. These could include objectively measurable events such as deaths, admissions or suicide attempts. Less objective outcomes, such as a decline in personal functioning, should be rated using a predetermined, reliable and valid scale. One should of course be open minded about unexpected differences between study groups, but these are hypothesis-generating rather than -confirming. Such serendipitous findings should be the focus of another study.

The rater should ideally apply the criteria in a blind manner, without knowing which group the patients belong to. Lack of blinding can bias the rater towards assigning the experimental group to poorer outcome ratings (unless the outcomes are very 'hard' events, such as death or admission). Even with good blinding raters may 'guess' the group membership of a patient through circumstantial evidence, such as the side effects of medication, the history of the patient, and even their rating scale scores.

In this paper criteria are indeed stated objectively: reconviction is the outcome of interest. Blinding is not necessary here because the reconviction details are obtained from the Offenders Index, which is (presumably) not influenced by the patients' diagnoses. It is important to remember, however, that not all offences may be detected, and that only a proportion of those detected will reach the conviction stage. Moreover, the Offenders Index records only serious offences. Other biases may apply as; for example, a mentally ill person may not be convicted for assault if he fulfils the criteria for an insanity plea. Mentally ill offenders are also sometimes admitted to hospital rather than tried, if they are acutely ill. Some patients may travel out of the area of the study, for example to another country, and may be equally likely to offend there without appearing in national records.

Question 5   Were corrections made for initial differences between or within groups? Were subgroups studied adequately?

When a study involves an experimental and a control cohort there may be important baseline differences between the groups (e.g. age, comorbid disorders, social class, etc.). These differences can influence the prognosis and will need to be controlled statistically.

Within a cohort there may be subgroups which are different from the rest of the group in some manner. These subgroups will need to be analysed separately to obtain an accurate picture of outcome and risks.

In this paper, correction for age, gender and any previous conviction has been attempted. Gender and destination on discharge were no longer associated with reconviction. Other factors (age at discharge, prior conviction and legal classification of psychopathic disorder) continued to be significant predictors of reconviction. Although the author found an association between the legal definition of psychopathic disorder and reconviction, it may have been informative to study some clinical factors as well (e.g. classification of psychotic illness, history of substance abuse, and perhaps specific descriptions of personality disorders). Such factors are considered important in predicting criminal behaviour clinically, and may have been adequately documented when the patient was admitted to the secure unit.

Question 6   Were these results validated in a test group?

If a cohort study identifies prognostic factors, it would be ideal if one could confirm these findings in another study. The confirmatory study should state explicitly that it will look for the influence of the prognostic factors as detected in the earlier study. This would rule out the influence of chance in showing some factors as prognostic. In practice these kinds of confirmation may come only with time as more studies are done. At other times a particular research group may combine data from various studies and report the overall risks.

Are the results important?

Assessing the importance of these results may be facilitated by displaying them in the form of a contingency table (Table 4.4).

Table 4.4   Conviction following discharge from a secure hospital setting

	Convicted (of total 425) %
Outcome after 5 years	24
Outcome after 10 years	31

Patients discharged from a state hospital therefore have a 24% probability of conviction in 5 years and 31% at 10 years. It does stand out that a relatively high proportion of the 425 patients discharged from the state hospital did reoffend. However, as there was no control group we do not know whether any psychiatric condition per se contributed to a high reconviction rate (but see Table 4.5). It would have been informative to contrast these figures with those of prison-discharged reoffenders.

Table 4.5 Contingency table showing the reconviction figures in those with mental illness, psychopathic disorders and mental impairment

	Reconvicted (of total 425) %
Mental illness (n = 190)	26
Psychopathic disorder (n = 141)	44
Mental impairment (n = 72)	32
Severe mental impairment (n = 45)	11

Question 1 What is the probability (or risk) of the outcomes over time?

For example, what is the relative risk of conviction in the presence of a psychopathic disorder rather than a mental illness?

The probability of reconviction in the presence of a psychopathic disorder is 0.44 (44%), and the probability of reconviction in the presence of a mental illness is 0.26 (26%).

Therefore,

$$\text{Relative risk} = \frac{\text{Risk of conviction in psychopathic cohort}}{\text{Risk of conviction in mentally ill cohort}}$$

$$= 0.44/0.26 = 1.69$$

A person with a legal definition of psychopathic disorder is likely to offend at 1.69 times the rate of a person with mental illness. This is quite high, as the baseline rate of offending is very high in this group.

Similar risk ratios could be calculated between other groups. The primary article uses odds ratios rather than risk ratios, probably because they can be produced by SPSS in the course of data analysis. Relative risks generally produce a more accurate estimate of risk than do odds ratios, especially where an event is common, as it is here.

Question 2 How precise are the prognosis estimates?

The confidence intervals can be calculated around a prognosis estimate. The unit used is usually the probability of an event occurring, and is estimated by the proportion of people (p) experiencing a given event. The standard error is calculated by:

$$\sqrt{\frac{p(1-p)}{n}}$$

where n is the sample size.

The confidence intervals for a proportion of people p experiencing an event is therefore:

$$p \pm 1.96 \times \text{standard error}$$

In our example 31% of all 425 discharged patients reoffend after 10 years: p is therefore 0.31, and the standard error for this estimate, from the above formula is:

$$\sqrt{\frac{0.31(1-0.31)}{425}} = 0.022 \ (2.2\%)$$

Therefore, the 95% confidence limits are

$$0.31 - 1.96 \times 0.022$$

to

$$0.31 + 1.96 \times 0.022$$

or

$$0.27 \ (27\%)$$

to

$$0.35 \ (35\%)$$

In other words, we can be 95% certain that the true probability of reoffending at 10 years is between 27 and 35% of all patients discharged from state hospital.

Can I apply these results to my patients?

Having found valid important evidence about prognosis, its usefulness to your particular clinical practice should now be considered. Two questions can help guide your judgement.

Question 1 Were the study patients similar to your own?

This involves assessing the similarity of your patients to those in the study in terms of the demographic characteristics and the setting.

You would like to know whether your patients are comparable with the patients in this study in terms of their index offences: this information is not provided in the paper. You work in a setting similar to that described in the paper; however, you would like to know more about the prognosis of specific mental disorders and whether specific symptoms predict criminality more strongly than others.

Question 2   Will the study alter your conclusions about what to offer or tell your patients?

If a prognosis study would make little impact on what you offer your patient(s) in terms of treatment or information, even valid important data would be of limited use. If the study informs you that an untreated disorder has a particularly poor prognosis, then you may be motivated to provide earlier effective treatment. However, if treatment is relatively ineffective and the prognosis is favourable, treatment may be justifiably withheld in some circumstances.

In this study the answers to this question are very interesting. To take just one example, 44% of patients with a legal category of psychopathic disorder have seriously reoffended 10 years after discharge from state hospital. They are 1.69 times as likely to do so as are patients in the category of mental illness. How does this influence us? Perhaps one conclusion would be that, even with treatment, psychopathically disordered individuals are likely to seriously reoffend; therefore, expensive state hospital treatment may not be justified and containment within the prison service is more suitable. Another interpretation might be that patients with psychopathic disorder are a particularly severely affected group who should be offered effective treatment as a priority. However, the question of whether such an effective treatment exists must be answered with the use of other evidence about the treatment of this disorder. Nevertheless, the information may be useful in providing advice to statutory agencies, such as the criminal justice system, as the probability of serious reoffending in these patients may influence the decision to give a hospital disposal and the degree of supervision offered in the community.

Conclusions

Having appraised the published article and found it to contain valid, important and clinically useful information, you present it to your local consultants. The evidence seems to add to the discussion in this controversial area, as most arguments are based on clinical experience and the personal opinions of various stakeholders. You resolve to supplement this study with a study of your own, aiming to examine whether certain types of psychiatric symptom are associated with serious reoffending.

Prognosis worksheet

Are the results of this prognosis study valid?

1. Was a defined, representative sample of patients assembled at a common (usually early) point in the course of their disease?

2. Was patient follow-up sufficiently long and complete?

3. Were objective outcome criteria applied in a 'blind' fashion?

4. If subgroups with different prognoses are identified, was there adjustment for important prognostic factors?

5. Was there validation in an independent group ('test-set') of patients?

Are the valid results of this prognosis study important?

1. How likely are the outcomes over time?

2. How precise are the prognostic estimates?

If you want to calculate a confidence interval around the measure of prognosis:

Clinical measure	Standard error (SE)
Number of patients = n Proportion of these patients who experience the event = p 95%CI = $P + 1.96 \times$ SE	$\sqrt{\{p \times (1 - p)/n\}}$

Can you apply this evidence about prognosis in caring for your patient?

1. Were the study patients similar to your own?

2. Will this evidence make a clinically important impact on your conclusions about what to offer or tell your patients?

META-ANALYSES AND SYSTEMATIC REVIEWS

Systematic reviews are comprehensive reviews of all the studies in a given area, which have been identified using explicit criteria. Meta-analysis is the statistical synthesis of the results derived from different research studies preferably located by a systematic review.

The results from a single study, no matter how well designed, are subject to systematic and unsystematic errors (i.e. bias and measurement errors). Ideally the results from a study need to be replicated several times, but study results will vary by chance and according to the precise methods used. One therefore commonly needs to aggregate the results from various studies which have a similar purpose and design. Weights are assigned to each study depending on its size or quality, so that large, high-quality studies will have greater bearing on the final results of the analysis.

Systematic reviews require an explicit method of searching several databases (e.g. MEDLINE, EMBASE, PsychLit), as well as examining references from any articles identified and hand searches of journals. Information can also be gathered by writing to experts in the field for unpublished data. Criteria for including and excluding studies should be explicitly framed before the search. The selected studies can also be ranked by preset criteria to assess their quality.

In general, a systematic review or meta-analysis may be critically appraised (Oxman et al 1994) under the following headings: Is the study valid? Are the results important? Can I use the study in caring for my patient(s)?

Clinical scenario

A 27-year-old man is admitted to the ward with a relapse of schizophrenia. His parents have heard that some of the newer antipsychotic drugs appear to be more effective in this condition. The consultants in your hospital are divided in their opinions about this. The parents particularly ask you about a drug called risperidone, as they have read about it on the Internet. As an interested trainee, you want to know whether there would be a great advantage in using this drug over the older drugs. The question here seems to be: what is the effectiveness of risperidone compared with traditional antipsychotics in treating schizophrenia in an adult male?

You search the Cochrane library CD-ROM in your hospital, identify the following paper and print it out to appraise it: 'Risperidone versus typical antipsychotic medication for schizophrenia' (Kennedy et al 1999).

Précis of published article

The authors carried out a comprehensive electronic search of various databases (MEDLINE, EMBASE, Biological Abstracts, PsychLit, SCISEARCH, Cochrane Schizophrenia Group Register and Cochrane Library), and references from these studies were searched for more citations. Randomized controlled trials comparing risperidone to any neuroleptic for the treatment of schizophrenia or any serious mental illness were selected. Twelve short-term and two long-term studies were identified and provided data on 3401 people. Odds ratios (OR), 95% confidence intervals (CI) and (where needed) the number needed to treat (NNT) were calculated on an intention-to-treat basis. Funnel plots showed that smaller studies showed greater benefit with risperidone. Risperidone increased the odds of improvement moderately (OR

1.54, CI 1.30 to 1.82; NNT 10, CI 7–16) but did not have a significant additional benefit on positive or negative symptoms. However, it did have less tendency to cause movement disorder, mainly in comparison with haloperidol (OR 0.43, CI 0.34–0.55; NNT 7, CI 5–10). Risperidone was slightly less likely to cause somnolence (OR 0.78, CI 0.61–0.99; NNT 22). Weight gain was more likely with risperidone (OR 1.51, CI 1.14–2.00; NNH 13). Sensitivity analysis with different doses of risperidone did not change the principal outcomes, but these were influenced by different doses of haloperidol.

Is this research valid?

Question 1   Did the study ask a clearly focused question?

A systematic review necessarily has to keep its question focused to be able to answer it reliably. An accompanying meta-analysis is a statistical summary of data from *similar* studies.

In this case the authors of the review state their objective to be the 'evaluation of effectiveness of risperidone for schizophrenia in comparison to conventional neuroleptic drugs'. This seems clear enough.

Question 2   Did the authors select the appropriate studies for the meta-analysis?

Meta-analysis can be used to address different areas of clinical interest, including aetiology, harm, diagnosis and, as in this example, treatment. The studies selected should have a design which is appropriate to the research issue. The authors need to state inclusion and exclusion selection criteria so as to reliably identify studies whose results can be effectively combined. A study of treatment efficacy is best addressed by using a randomized controlled trial design. In this example the authors identified 14 relevant randomized controlled trials.

Question 3   What did the authors do to rule out bias in the selection of studies?

Bias in a systematic review can arise from several sources. Language bias usually arises by focusing on English-language articles, thereby missing out possibly important publications in other languages. In practice these are usually small negative studies, and language bias is usually a form of publication bias. Publication bias arises because journals accept and receive more articles which have a positive finding. Multiple publication of the same data can be hard to detect, but can be another important source of publication bias. Funnel plot analysis is one way of identifying publication bias, by plotting the precision (i.e. the inverse of the standard error) against a measure of effect size (e.g. the log of the odds ratio, the effect size statistic, etc.). The precision is plotted on the y (ordinate) axis and the effect size is plotted on the x (abscissa) axis (see Chapter 3 for an example). In the absence of publication bias smaller studies will be scattered around the top and larger studies will aggregate at the bottom, to give a funnel shape. A positive publication bias can be identified by an absence of small negative studies.

A Galbraith plot can be adapted to generate a P value for publication bias. The two measures used are the 'standard normal deviate (SND)', which is the log odds divided by the standard error, and the 'precision', which is the inverse of the standard error. These are fitted into a linear regression equation of the form

$$SND = a + b \times precision$$

On a graph smaller studies will be close to zero on both the axes. This is because small studies will have large standard errors and therefore the values of both the SND and precision will be relatively small. Larger studies will have smaller standard errors and the SND will be closer to the true effect size. Stated simply, the regression line will not pass through the origin in the presence of a publication bias and the 90% confidence interval of this intercept gives the P value for publication bias.

The authors of the risperidone review conducted a funnel plot analysis and concluded that negative outcome studies may not have been published. Thus, the results are likely to be influenced by a publication bias in favour of risperidone.

Question 4   How were the relevant studies located?

A systematic search strategy must be detailed before the relevant studies are sought out. Normally, electronic databases are searched using a defined search strategy, and identified studies may have references to other studies, which should also be obtained. A painstaking hand search of important journals, going back several years, is also required. Writing to experts, research groups and pharmaceutical companies should also be undertaken, in an attempt to include unpublished trial data in the analysis.

The authors of the review conducted electronic searches of the Cochrane Schizophrenia Group Register, Biological Abstracts, EMBASE, MEDLINE, PsychLit and SCISEARCH. The selected studies were searched to identify more references. Pharmaceutical companies and researchers in the area were contacted for unpublished studies. This is a systematic and comprehensive search.

Question 5   Did the reviewers assess the quality of the studies? Did they use a description of randomization and/or a rating scale?

Ideally, objective criteria for rating the studies, on the basis of randomization, blinding and intention-to-treat analysis, should be used by more than one rater. The raters should be blind to the source and authors of the studies. An interrater reliability should be calculated to check how similar the raters' assessments are. There should be a specified way to reach a consensus in case of disagreements between the ratings of the different raters.

The authors of this systematic review have a specified way of rating the studies using three raters, but the actual procedure for rating has not been made explicit. It is not clear whether an objective rating scale was used, or whether the ratings were done with adequate blinding. The authors do, however, grade the trials into classes A and B, on the basis of whether they describe how they concealed the randomization or not. They also describe how they settled disagreements between raters.

What are the results?

Question 1   Are the results clearly displayed?

There is a tabular display of results in Cochrane reviews called a 'metaview'. The dark diamonds represent the point estimation of effect for each study, which in this example is an odds ratio. The lozenges represent pooled odds ratios. This is a weighted average of odds ratios from all the selected studies. Odds ratios or any measure of effect size can be weighted by using standard errors. The smaller the standard error in a study, the more weight it is assigned. The horizontal lines represent the 95% confidence interval, with their ends anchored at the 95% confidence limits.

Odds ratios are used when studies have dichotomous outcomes, such as 'alive' or 'dead', 'improved' or 'not improved'. When a continuous measure like a rating scale is used there are two ways of analysing the resulting data: the outcomes can be converted to dichotomous categories by setting an arbitrary cut-off – for example, a 20% decrease in scores could be regarded as an improvement – and then calculating odds ratios; alternatively, the data can also be analysed as a continuous variable and overall effect size calculated as a 'weighted mean difference'.

Question 2   Were the results from various studies different, and what explains any variation?

Basic differences in methodology, e.g. sampling, types of subject and differences in intervention, could account for differences between studies. Usually the reviewer carries out statistical procedures called tests of heterogeneity to detect such differences at the outset. Statistically significant heterogeneity of treatment effects implies that the difference between the results of the studies could not have arisen by chance, i.e. there is heterogeneity, and calculating a single summary effect size may be unreliable. However, a lack of significant heterogeneity does not rule out inherent differences amongst the studies as the heterogeneity test has low power. In our example, there is no heterogeneity, i.e. the studies had similar outcomes.

Question 3   What is the overall result of the review?

The results will depend on the measures used and the outcomes studied. The studies in this review focused on clinical improvement rating scales and the measurement of side effects. The PANSS was used by nine studies and we will focus on this here.

Normally, summary results are calculated in terms of ORs, ARRs or ABIs and NNTs, with confidence intervals. Studies in this systematic review used different cut-offs for improvement to depict outcome in a dichotomous manner. These ranged from 20

Table 4.6   Data from nine studies in the form of a contingency (2 × 2) table

	Improved %	Not improved %
'Typical drug'	53	47
Risperidone	42	58

to 60% reduction on the PANSS scores, but nine studies used 20%. An intention-to-treat analysis was used to take dropouts into account.

From Table 4.6:

$$ABI = 53 - 42 = 11\%$$

$$NNT = 100/11 = 9.1 \text{ (CI } 7\text{--}16)$$

$$OR = 47 \times 42/53 \times 58 = 0.65 \text{ (CI } 0.55\text{--}0.77)$$

NB: Cochrane reviews tend to report all positive (desirable) outcomes as less than 1, and vice versa, such that this means the odds of not improving are reduced by 0.65 on risperidone (or that the odds of improving are 1/0.65 = 1.54). The confidence intervals for these calculations are shown within brackets. Note there is a wide range for the NNT value. An NNT of 9.1 means that 10 'whole' patients need to be treated with risperidone to get one patient better, compared with standard medication. As the confidence interval is wide the NNT may well be higher than 10. Note that improvement has been defined as a 20% reduction in PANSS scores, which may not be a remarkable difference in clinical terms. Moreover, we already know that the trials here suffer from publication bias, and that negative trials may have been underreported. Overall, therefore, the gains of risperidone in terms of improved efficacy in treating psychotic symptoms are not impressive. However, the results for extrapyramidal side effects are more promising.

Eight studies provided data and overall they favour risperidone (OR 0.43, NNT 5, CI 5–10), i.e. five individuals need to be treated with risperidone to prevent one person from experiencing a drug-induced movement disorder.

The effects of different doses of medications on outcome has been examined with a sensitivity analysis. The outcome of studies does not change radically with different doses of risperidone, but when data from studies using >10 mg of haloperidol are omitted, risperidone turns out to be less effective but retains an advantage in terms of reducing the odds of movement disorders. The advantages of risperidone may therefore be more marked in patients on high doses of haloperidol, and relatively few in those on low doses.

Can I apply these results in treating my patient(s)?

Question 1 Do these figures apply to my patients?

This study incorporates data from different centres and probably different clinical practice conditions. The results probably therefore apply to your patients.

Question 2 How great will be the potential benefit to your patient?

The NNT calculated for a modest improvement of 20% in PANSS scores is 10 in this analysis. The baseline rate of improvement of your patients using the outcomes in your clinical practice is called the PEER. If your patients have a better chance of improvement on standard drugs, rather than those in the study, risperidone is likely to be of less value to them. However, if your patients were more susceptible to the side effects than were those in this review, risperidone may be worth considering. These relative benefits can be calculated using a PEER, or estimated with *F*, as already described in the previous section on treatment.

Question 3 Will this treatment agree with the values and preferences of your patient?

This question should be asked only if the study has met both the scientific validity and the clinical importance criteria. It is, however, obvious that most patients would want a more effective treatment with fewer side effects.

Conclusions

The review shows modest benefits of risperidone but there appears to be a publication bias in favour of risperidone. You therefore surmise that risperidone cannot be recommended over a traditional drug, based on current knowledge, unless the patient has unacceptable extrapyramidal side effects.

Although this is not a paper on economic analysis, the authors do comment on the significant cost of risperidone over traditional drugs. This should also be a part of decision making for treatment.

Systematic review worksheet

Is the study valid?

Is it a systematic review of randomized trials of the treatment you're interested in?

Does it include a methods section that describes:
- finding and including all the relevant trials?

- assessing their individual validity?

Were the results consistent from study to study?

Are the results important?

Translating odds ratios to NNTs. The numbers in the body of the table are the NNTs for the corresponding odds ratios at that particular patient's expected event rate (PEER).

		Odds Ratios (OR)								
		0.9	0.85	0.8	0.75	0.7	0.65	0.6	0.55	0.5
	0.05	209	139	104	83	69	59	52	46	41
Patient	0.10	110	73	54	43	36	31	27	24	21
expected	0.20	61	40	30	24	20	17	14	13	11
event	0.30	46	30	22	18	14	12	10	9	8
rate	0.40	40	26	19	15	12	10	9	8	7
(PEER)	0.50	38	25	18	14	11	9	8	7	6
	0.70	44	28	20	16	13	10	9	7	6
	0.90	101	64	46	34	27	22	18	15	12

Can you apply the results in caring for your patient?

Do these results apply to your patient?

Is your patient so different from those in
the overview that its results can't help
you?

How great would the potential benefit of
therapy actually be for your individual
patient?

Method 1: In the table above, find the intersection of the closest odds ratio from the
overview and your patient's expected event rate if they received the control
treatment (PEER):

Method 2: to calculate the NNT for any OR and PEER:

$$NNT = \frac{1-[PEER \times (1-OR)]}{(1-PEER) \times PEER \times (1-OR)}$$

Can I use this systematic review in caring for my patient(s)?

Do you and your patient have a clear
assessment of their values and
preferences?

Are they met by this regimen and its
consequences?

Should you believe apparent qualitative differences in the efficacy of therapy in some
subgroups of patients? Only if you can say 'yes' to all of the following:

1. Do they really make biologic and clinical sense?

2. Is the qualitative difference both clinically (beneficial for some but useless or
   harmful for others) and statistically significant?

3. Was this difference hypothesized before the study began (rather than the product
   of dredging the data), and has it been confirmed in other, independent studies?

4. Was this one of just a few subgroup analyses carried out in this study?

ECONOMIC EVALUATION

Economic analysis aims to take a wider perspective on healthcare provision. The NHS has limited economic resources and it is important to use them in a way that maximizes the total healthcare benefit. Money may be used to purchase employees, drugs, investigations, beds or even hospitals. Their benefits may be measured in the benefit they bring to patients in terms of outcome, but there may also be benefits to society as a whole. The costs of providing a resource may have costs to individuals, for example in terms of side effects, but also has financial costs to society as a whole. The task of taking into account all the potential costs and benefits and making an evaluation is the role of economic analysis. The critical appraisal of an article on economic evaluation follows the same three major questions as before (Drummond et al 1997b, O'Brien et al 1997), starting with 'Is the study valid?'. The second question, 'Is the study important?', is answered for an economic study by looking at the clinically relevant data, the most common being measures of cost-effectiveness, cost–benefit or cost–utility (see below). The third and last question is 'Can I use this study in caring for my patients?'.

Clinical scenario

You attend the board meeting of your general hospital to discuss clinical interventions for the treatment of schizophrenia. There is considerable scepticism about the routine use of clozapine in patients with treatment-resistant schizophrenia. Some argue that the money would be better spent elsewhere, for example on counselling for depression. You are nominated to undertake a literature review and find a Canadian article covering specifically this area (Glennie 1997). You decide to appraise this article critically.

Précis of published article

This economic evaluation compares clozapine with haloperidol (HAL) and chlorpromazine (CPZ) in the treatment of hospitalized treatment-resistant schizophrenic patients with positive symptoms. The paper takes a government payer perspective and uses a cost–utility analysis as its overall approach. Direct costs, of medical treatment only, were considered. A decision model was adopted based on a literature review and expert consensus. The basis of this approach is, having chosen a treatment, to calculate the probabilities and consequences of each possible downstream event based on the published literature. Such events included 'success', 'failure', discharge from hospital and relapse. For outcomes without available data in the literature, an expert consensus arrived at an estimate. Costs and outcomes were evaluated over 1 year and projected over a lifetime. Future costs and outcomes were discounted at a rate of 5% (i.e. 'inflation' was calculated as 5% per annum). The evaluation then makes a number of assumptions about the doses of medication, frequency of blood monitoring, efficacy and life expectancy. Health state utilities were then obtained using a standard gamble technique and rating scale (a method where patients indicate their preferences for chronic health states by deciding whether they are preferable to or worse than death). Interviews were carried out with seven schizophrenic patients whom the clinic nurse felt would sufficiently understand the various outcome scenarios. The results given are the expected annual costs and outcomes for patients treated with clozapine compared to those treated with HAL/CPZ. The total annual costs per patient treated with clozapine were $90,727 (Canadian), with a utility rating of 0.86, whereas, for HAL/CPZ the annual costs were $129,607 with a utility rating of 0.82. Clozapine was therefore concluded to be the dominant therapy as it was associated with the lowest overall cost and the highest number of quality-adjusted life years. A number of one-way sensitivity analyses were carried out as part of the study, where costs were varied from 50% to 150% of baseline, and probability and utility values were carried from 0 to 1. None of the changes in cost variables altered the study conclusions, and variations in the probability and utility estimates only threatened the conclusions if utility ratings lay outside the 95% confidence interval or if the efficacy of clozapine fell to that of chlorpromazine.

Is the study valid?

Question 1 Does the study compare well defined and alternative courses of action?

Economic analyses always compare the costs and consequences of two or more courses of action. In some circumstances the alternative action may be no intervention at all, but more usually, for ethical reasons, economic studies will compare two active interventions alongside each other. This may be conducted alongside a randomized controlled trial, or alternatively the economic data may be derived from separate sources. In either case it is important that the alternative courses of action are clearly and explicitly defined. This point is very important in economic analysis, as a central concept is that of **opportunity cost**. Opportunity cost is the lack of resources to do something else: resources used in one way mean that the benefits of another intervention are foregone.

The current study of treatment-resistant schizophrenia compares clozapine with the antipsychotics chlorpromazine and haloperidol. These were selected as they are commonly used and are the least expensive alternatives to clozapine.

Question 2   Does the study take a well specified, preferably broad, viewpoint?

Economic analyses may take a variety of viewpoints. Hospital- or trust-based viewpoints deal with the costs and benefits locally, but ignore the benefits and costs to society as a whole. The widest possible viewpoint is preferable if all the costs and benefits of a manoeuvre are to be accounted for.

The current study uses a 'government payer perspective'. It could have taken a broader perspective, for example that of society as a whole, but claims that it could not do this because insufficient information was available. Many important costs will not have been considered, for example the costs to the individuals concerned and the local community. These non-medical costs (of time off work, reduced productivity, etc.) are sometimes called **indirect costs**.

Question 3   Does the study use clinically useful expressions of the costs and consequences of alternative courses of clinical action?

Studies citing evidence for the cost and consequences of a certain action must use clinically useful expressions if their conclusions are to be of use to clinicians. **Cost-effectiveness analysis** measures health benefits in natural units, such as life years saved, or by improvements on a rating scale. The cost-effectiveness ratio is the major unit used in these studies, derived by dividing the costs of these interventions by their healthcare benefit. Different interventions must therefore be comparable in terms of the unit of healthcare benefit. **Cost–utility analysis** measures a healthcare intervention's effect on both quality and quantity of life. Healthcare effects are converted into utilities (health state preference scores, 1 being optimum health quality and 0 being no subjective health quality at all), usually generating a cost per quality-adjusted life year gained (QALY). The principles are similar to cost-effectiveness analysis in that the major unit of analysis used for the comparison of 'cost–utility' is the ratio of cost number to QALYs gained. Healthcare interventions with different outcomes (or even different interventions) can be converted into the same units with this type of analysis, whereas they could not be analysed with a cost-effectiveness analysis. Finally, **cost–benefit analysis** converts all the costs and consequences of a healthcare intervention into the same units, usually monetary. Different interventions can be compared, even when the outcomes are very different.

This study uses the QALY as a measure of treatment efficacy. This is an often-used clinical measure that takes into account not only the life years gained, but also their relative quality. Thus years rated by patients as having a high quality of life are rated more favourably than those rated as having a low, or less favourable, quality.

Question 4 Does the study cite good evidence on the accuracy and efficacy of alternatives?

Economic analyses tend to assume that the effects of different manoeuvres are highly predictable. In order to be comfortable with this assumption, one must be satisfied that the evidence leading to that decision is reliable. For example, a cost-effectiveness analysis of two drugs should preferably cite randomized controlled evidence of their comparative efficacies, if not information from a meta-analysis. Non-experimental evidence and open-label studies are less likely to provide accurate evidence of efficacy. However, studies such as RCTs, although they have high internal validity, may be less generalizable to clinical practice. Pragmatic trials, which study how effective an intervention is in clinical practice, are likely to be more generalizable to clinical practice but more susceptible to bias. Such studies are said to have greater external validity but less internal validity.

The current study cites evidence from three randomized controlled trials comparing clozapine with either chlorpromazine or haloperidol. The authors claim that 'standard meta-analysis methods' were used. They do not state whether all relevant articles were identified, how they were evaluated, and whether the results were similar from study to study. Their methodology cannot therefore be scrutinized and may be flawed.

Question 5 Does the study identify all of the costs and benefits that you think it should, and select credible measures for them?

All the costs and benefits of a course of action should be identified by a study. They should include all the costs to the organization and individuals supplying the care and all the costs and benefits to those receiving the care. The terms direct and indirect costs are sometimes used in this context. **Direct costs** are the resources consumed by the programme rather than an alternative. These costs would usually be resources in the healthcare sector, but would sometimes include patients' 'out-of-pocket' expenses and costs from other statutory and voluntary agencies. **Indirect costs**, on the other hand, are productivity gains and losses. The focus is usually on patient time consumed or freed up by the healthcare programme. Sometimes the term is used to refer to overhead costs (e.g. light, heat, rental or capital costs), especially by the accountancy profession. Direct and indirect costs are, however, inconsistently used terms and one should always carefully examine the exact nature of any costs.

The study considers only the costs to government. Indirect costs, such as gains or losses in patient productivity, were not considered. This is a limitation to the study.

Is the study important?

Question 1 Are the resulting costs or costs per unit health gained impressive?

The effects of a manoeuvre may be measured in three main ways, each with a specific method of interpretation.

Cost-effectiveness analysis

Effects may be measured in a common unit of cost per healthcare gain. Such measures may include cost per life year gained, costs per remission achieved, etc., in a 'cost-effectiveness' analysis.

Each treatment, or management strategy, is compared with an alternative in terms of the cost per unit of healthcare gained. If a treatment is more effective at the same or less cost than an alternative, the interpretation is simple. However, if a more expensive and more effective treatment is compared with an existing treatment, the interpretation of the data is less straightforward. In these circumstances the term **incremental cost** is used. This is the additional cost per unit of healthcare gained by switching from the less to the more expensive therapy.

Cost–utility analysis

Examining the social value of different interventions is an alternative way of comparing outcome. The consumers of healthcare interventions are central to this approach. The measure includes not only the years of life gained but also the relative quality of that life to the individual. The unit used is sometimes referred to as a quality-adjusted life year (QALY). This method lends itself to 'cost–utility' analysis, in which management strategies are compared in terms of the cost per QALY gained. Individual therapies are often compared in terms of the cost per QALY to a league table of other treatments available in the hospital. However, the incremental cost per QALY is also used and the principles are very similar to those of cost-effectiveness analysis (Table 4.7).

Table 4.7 Hypothetical table of cost per QALY gained

Treatment	Cost/QALY (£)
Hip replacement	1100
β-Interferon for multiple sclerosis	500 000
Imipramine for depression	8000

The reader should be aware that there are major limitations to the use of a so-called cost-effectiveness 'league table'. The methodology of the studies cited in the table must be sound and relatively homogeneous from study to study: 'league tables' may also mislead in deciding which healthcare intervention to choose. The interested reader may like to read the texts by Drummond et al (1997a,b).

Cost–benefit analysis

Outcomes may be converted to a common unit of currency for comparison. This method raises some conceptual difficulties, as it may require the value of a life, for example, to be stated in monetary terms. This type of data lends itself to 'cost–benefit' analysis.

Treatments are then compared with each other in terms of the common unit of money. This type of analysis has become less popular than cost-effectiveness analysis in recent years.

The current study examines healthcare utilities (QALYs) as a measure of healthcare benefit comparatively for two treatments. It is therefore a cost–utility analysis, although some researchers, particularly in the USA, would not distinguish this study from a cost-effectiveness study that uses utilities as its outcome measure. The study does not give the cost per QALY gained, although this figure may be calculated from the results. The study states that $39,000 of savings are made per year with clozapine rather than with chlorpromazine and haloperidol, while producing 0.04 more QALYs. In a later table it goes on to give the expected annual costs and outcomes for clozapine. The expected QALYs gained over 1 year with clozapine are approximately 0.86 at a cost of approximately $90,727, a cost per QALY of $105,497. At the time of writing this is a cost per QALY of £43,852. This compares well with interferon treatment in our hypothetical league table, but poorly with hip replacement and imipramine for depression. However, as clozapine achieves greater healthcare benefit than chlorpromazine, and more cheaply, it can be concluded that it is the dominant therapy in this study. Cost per QALY gained is generally much higher for chronic illnesses such as schizophrenia.

Question 2   Are the conclusions unlikely to change with sensible changes in costs and outcomes?

Whatever the results of an economic analysis, the statement of a single conclusion without further qualification is unwarranted. Clinical practice is unlikely to mimic exactly the conditions of the analysis, and therefore the effect of uncertainty on the conclusions of the study must be considered. The study must state whether it has examined its conclusions in such a way as to account for sensible variations in costs and outcomes that would take place in clinical practice. This important approach is referred to as sensitivity analysis, and can be divided into three main types (Briggs 1999): one-way, extreme scenario and Monte Carlo. A one-way sensitivity analysis measures the effect of changing each variable in the study across a plausible range of values while keeping all other parameters constant. An extreme scenario sensitivity analysis involves setting each variable at its most optimistic or pessimistic value while holding the others constant. However, as variables rarely change in isolation, one-way analyses tend to underestimate the uncertainty in an economic evaluation, and extreme scenario analyses tend to overestimate the uncertainty. This has led to a third type of sensitivity analysis known as probabilistic, or 'Monte Carlo'. This examines the effects of simultaneously varying a number of the study's underlying parameters across a predefined range, according to a predefined distribution. This type of analysis is expected to produce a more realistic measure of a study's uncertainty.

The current study performs a number of one-way sensitivity analyses. Cost parameters are varied from 50% to 150% of baseline, whereas probability and utility values are varied from 0 to 1. Threshold values – the point at which the conclusions of the analysis shifted from one strategy to the other – were determined for all key parameters used in the analysis. None of the changes in cost variable affected the rank ordering of the expected costs. Chlorpromazine became the optimal therapy only when utilities reached values outside their 95% confidence interval, as defined for the various scenarios. The sensitivity analysis also suggested that if the success rate for clozapine became the same as for chlorpromazine, chlorpromazine would become the more cost-effective therapy. This was thought to be unlikely because of the evidence from randomized controlled trials, and because treatment-resistant patients were, by definition, resistant to standard therapy.

Can I use the study in caring for my patients?

Having decided that an economic analysis contains both valid and important information on a manoeuvre, how can you decide whether it should be adopted as a strategy? The following questions may act as a useful guide.

Question 1 Do the costs apply in my setting?

The economic costs may not apply directly to your setting, as resources may have different costs and availabilities in your current practice.

The current study is conducted in Canada, where the costs of medication and healthcare provision are likely to be different from those in the UK. The doubt that remains cannot be addressed without conducting a cost of illness study in this country.

Question 2   Are the interventions likely to be as effective in your setting?

When critically appraising an article on therapy or diagnosis it is important to consider how the intervention would behave in your environment. If the benefits of a manoeuvre are not realized, the economic analysis may not apply to your setting.

The current study compares the efficacy of clozapine in treatment-resistant schizophrenia compared with chlorpromazine and haloperidol. Haloperidol is used less often in the UK than in the US. However, the indications for clozapine are similar in both countries, and it is unlikely that there would be a substantial effect on the comparative clinical efficacy of each treatment.

Question 3   Is it worth it?

Having appraised the evidence from an economic analysis and found both valid and important evidence for a manoeuvre, what factors should be considered when deciding whether or not to adopt it? The answer depends on the question being asked.

If a cost-minimization analysis has been performed, where the outcomes are the same but the costs differ, is the difference in cost worth switching to the cheaper therapy? Other factors would have to be taken into account such as administrative reorganization and disruption to others. If a cost–utility analysis has been performed, where does the intervention lie on the local league table? If a cost-effectiveness analysis has been performed, is the difference in cost sufficient to make you want to spend that difference (where a greater effect is achieved at an equal or lower cost)? Or, if a more effective treatment is available at a greater cost, does the incremental cost justify expanding your treatment to the more expensive one?

Although the current study examines the cost–utility of clozapine in terms of cost per QALY, it also uses this measure comparatively as a measure of cost-effectiveness. The cost per QALY for clozapine is substantial but less than other treatments on our league table, for example β-interferon. Furthermore, using QALYs as a measure, clozapine is more cost-effective than conventional antipsychotic drugs for the management of treatment-resistant schizophrenia.

Conclusions

The above is a brief guide to the critical appraisal of an economic analysis. Other types of less commonly used study have not been covered and the interested reader should read the other texts (Jefferson et al 1996, Drummond et al 1997a & b) given at the end of this chapter.

Economic analysis worksheet

Is the study valid?

1. Is this report really asking an economic question:

- Comparing well defined alternative courses of action?

- With a specified point of view (a hospital, a ministry of health, or preferably society as a whole) from which the costs and effects are being viewed?

- With clinically useful expressions of the costs and consequences of the alternative courses of clinical action?

- Effects equal, and a simple comparison of costs: cost-minimization analysis.

- Effects unequal but measured in the same common unit of health: cost-effectiveness analysis.

- Effects both unequal and measured in more than one kind of unit of health:
  - converted into monetary units: cost–benefit analysis.
  - converted into personal preferences or utilities (QALYs): cost–utility analysis.

---

2. Does it cite good evidence (that would meet the therapy, diagnosis, or overview guides) on the efficacy/accuracy of the alternatives?

---

3. Does it identify all the costs and effects you think it should, and did it select credible measures for them?

Are the valid results important?

1. Are the resulting costs or costs/unit of
   health gained impressive?

2. Are the conclusions unlikely to change
   with sensible changes in costs and
   outcomes?

A 'league table' of costs to gain one additional quality-adjusted life
year (QALY) (from Drummond et al 1997a):

Treatment	Cost/QALY (£ Aug 1990)
Neurosurgical intervention for head injury	240
Advice to stop smoking from general practitioner	270
Valve replacement for aortic stenosis	1140
Coronary artery bypass graft (left main vessel disease, severe angina)	2090
Breast cancer screening	5780
Cholesterol testing and treatment (incrementally) of all adults aged 25–39	14,150
Continuous ambulatory peritoneal dialysis	19,870
Hospital haemodialysis	21,970
Erythropoietin treatment for anaemia in dialysis patients (assuming 10% reduction in mortality)	54,380
Neurosurgical intervention for malignant intracranial tumours	107,780
Erythropoietin treatment for anaemia in dialysis patients (assuming no increase in survival)	126,290

Can I use this study in caring for my patient(s)?

1. Do the costs in it apply in your own setting?
2. Are the treatments likely to be as effective in your setting?
3. Is it worth it?
• If a cost-minimization analysis, is the difference in costs big enough to warrant switching over to the cheaper therapy?
• If a cost-effectiveness analysis, is the difference in effectiveness great enough for you to want to spend the difference?
• If a cost–utility analysis, where does it lie in your local, current league table?

CLINICAL GUIDELINES

Clinical guidelines are becoming increasingly important and numerous. Despite this, there should be scepticism as to whether they are useful and about the motives of those who publish them. Where clinical practice varies widely, guidelines may be particularly useful in helping to provide patients with the best level of care, and also in minimizing costs. The critical appraisal of a clinical guideline follows the three now familiar questions (Hayward et al 1995, Wilson et al 1995). The first asks 'Is the guideline valid?'. The second question, 'Is the guideline important?', is answered by looking at the likely changes in clinical practice and the costs that would result from its adoption. The third and last question is 'Can I use this guidline in caring for my patients?', and is the final step before applying guidelines in your clinical practice.

Clinical scenario

You are a consultant in the psychiatry of old age in a busy urban hospital, with one acute admission and four long-stay wards to cover. You are becoming increasingly concerned that demented patients are routinely prescribed thioridazine when their behaviour becomes difficult to control, and that this medication is continued for a considerable length of time after the problem behaviour has settled. Clinical practice in this area varies widely, particularly within your own hospital. A colleague brings to your attention a clinical practice guideline that has recently been published in this area (SIGN 1998). You wonder whether this guideline may be useful and decide to critically appraise it, along with other members of the multidisciplinary team.

Précis of published article

The guideline, recommended for use in Scotland, is a 26-page document which can only be briefly summarized here. The guideline development group consisted of consultant psychiatrists, fieldworkers, pharmacists, nurses, psychologists, geriatricians, social workers and user groups (Alzheimer's Scotland). The interventions considered were pharmacological (neuroleptic and non-neuroleptic) and non-pharmacological (psychological and behaviourally based) therapies. The latter included reality orientation, behavioural intervention, occupational activities, environmental modifications, validation therapy, reminiscence and sensory stimulation. Outcomes of interest included restlessness, overactivity, mood disturbance, anxiety, depression, irritability, psychotic symptoms, disordered communication, repetitive noisiness, aggression and sexual disinhibition. A systematic review was undertaken for the guideline, covering 'an assessment of interventions in the management of behavioural and psychological aspects of dementia'. Although precise search terms were not specified, MEDLINE, EMBASE and Psychological abstracts and the Cochrane database were searched. The search terms were a list of psychiatric and behavioural symptoms, a range of psychotropic drugs, psychological treatments and behavioural modifications. The shortlisted papers were reviewed in detail and graded according to AHCPR (US Agency for Health Care Policy and Research) levels of evidence. The guideline also includes a summary of its findings and a single-sheet quick-reference guide.

Is the guideline valid?

To determine whether a clinical practice guideline is valid or not, it is useful to ask yourself several questions about the methodology used by those who submitted it for publication. If the guideline was formed on the basis of insufficient evidence, there is no need to discuss the article any further as the recommendations are likely to be biased.

Question 1   Were all important management decisions, options and outcomes clearly stated?

Whether a guideline is formed to steer practice in the field of treatment, diagnosis or prevention, its content will refer to the different choices available and their potential consequences. To appreciate why a particular action has been recommended, you must check that the developers have considered all the important outcomes and consequences available before deciding whether to subsequently reject or accept them. For example, a guideline on the treatment of schizophrenia that did not consider the use of clozapine would be seriously flawed.

The clinical practice guideline we have decided to appraise considers all the common options. It also extends its remit to many other treatments, both pharmacological and non-pharmacological, that are not routinely used in clinical practice.

Question 2   Was all the evidence relevant to each decision option identified, validated and combined sensibly and explicitly?

If, having successfully identified all the important options and outcomes, you wish to weight the recommendations of the guideline sensibly, an extensive search for the consequences of each action must be undertaken. Contributors must be careful not to bias the results of the guideline by citing evidence selectively. In effect, they must have access to, or carry out, a systematic review of that area. An exhaustive attempt must be made to search the literature for any articles of potential relevance to the guideline. Having identified articles, there must then be an explicit and reproducible method for weighting their results according to quality or precision. For example, when a guideline recommending treatments is formed, a well conducted meta-analysis with little or no heterogeneity is accepted as the highest recommendation (Table 4.8). Large randomized controlled trials, open trials and other experimental studies can also be considered, in decreasing order of importance. Case reports or consensus statements offer the least reliable type of evidence on which to base a clinical practice guideline.

Table 4.8 Levels of evidence associated with a therapeutic recommendation

Level of evidence	Therapeutic study
Ia	Meta-analysis of randomized controlled trials
Ib	Individual RCT
IIa	Well designed non-randomized controlled studies
IIb	Other well designed quasi-experimental studies
III	Evidence from well designed non-experimental studies
IV	Evidence from expert committee reports and experience of respected authorities

In the guideline we are considering an extensive literature search was made of several databases, including EMBASE, MEDLINE, Psychological abstracts and Cochrane, but the precise search terms are not stated. The shortlisted papers were reviewed 'in detail' using AHCPR levels of evidence, which cite meta-analyses as the highest level of evidence and the recommendations of expert committees as the lowest. Grades of recommendation were then made using this hierarchy of evidence as a guide, using an explicit method stated inside the front cover of the document.

Question 3   Are the benefits, costs and risks of each outcome considered from the perspective of different stakeholders?

Despite representation from a broad range of perspectives and disciplines the recommendations of a clinical guideline may be unduly influenced by the views of one panel member. One way to overcome this potential bias is to consider all the available perspectives using a structured and explicit system. It is particularly important in the development of guidelines that the patient perspective is taken into account and, where there is disagreement or ambivalence in values, that these are acknowledged.

In the current example, views were canvassed from a wide range of disciplines and perspectives. Medical, nursing, paramedical and user groups were all consulted. It is not, however, stated whether systematic and explicit methods were used to consider all perspectives. This may have led to bias being introduced, or to ambivalence or disagreement being unresolved/unacknowledged. It would have been better methodologically to have structured procedures in place.

Question 4   Is the guideline resistant to clinically sensible variations in practice?

The outcomes of the various recommendations contained in a guideline may, in practice, vary from the environment in which the guideline was validated. If the guideline is not valid for your patients, even if there are only minor deviations from the treatment efficacy quoted in the paper you may wish to dispense with it.

The guideline seems to cite a wide variety of evidence from different sources, and many clinicians from backgrounds similar to your own have been represented. It is unlikely that clinically sensible variations in practice would invalidate its recommendations.

Is the guideline important?

Question 1   Is there currently a large variation in clinical practice?

Guidelines are particularly helpful where there is a large variation in clinical practice that could be remedied by the introduction of a quality-improving strategy. Clinician practice may vary widely for many reasons, but if the best evidence is being used the variation should not be significant. In your experience other clinical teams may deal with the treatment of behavioural disturbance very differently. However, if clinical practice in your own hospital varies less, there being, perhaps, a generally heavy reliance (or not) on medication to treat behavioural problems of this kind, a guideline could still be useful if, for example, medication is not (or is) generally suitable.

Question 2   Does the guideline contain new evidence, or old evidence not yet acted upon, that could affect management?

The delay between the publication of new evidence and its adoption is often considerable. Clearly, clinical guidelines can aid clinical practice if they contain new evidence, or old evidence not yet acted upon.

In our example there appears to be a great deal of relatively recent evidence supporting psychological therapies. There is also a relative lack of evidence to support the long-term use of medication.

Question 3 Would the guideline have major effects on health outcome?

Where guidelines recommend effective treatments where before there were none, the implications for patient care could be very great. However, where small changes can be made in a large number of patients, or where large differences are made in a few high-risk patients, the changes in clinical outcome may also be significant.

In our example new ways of managing behavioural problems in dementia could have a major impact on a large number of people, as dementia is a very common condition. Furthermore, if the practice of antipsychotic prescription could be somewhat curtailed, there is evidence that the harm done to patients with dementia could be reduced.

Question 4 Would the guideline have major effects on resources?

Where a guideline recommends new, expensive treatments the effects on resources may be considerable. Guidelines may reduce as well as increase costs to hospitals, or even to society as a whole. For example, if the prescription of a new expensive therapy meant more patients returned to work, the new treatment would be cost-effective but place a major strain on hospital resources. It is important also to bear in mind the concept of opportunity cost here, where for any intervention used there is another action foregone.

Can I use this guideline in caring for my patients?

Question 1 What barriers are there to its implementation?

Guideline development usually takes place in an environment which is (at least in some ways) dissimilar to your own workplace. Such differences may invalidate the guideline, but more commonly there will be significant differences that need to be addressed before the guideline can be successfully implemented.

In our example there are major implications for the provision of psychological therapies, for which staff are not currently trained.

You estimate that new staff will need to be recruited, and that extra financial resources will be needed.

Question 2   Can you enlist the collaboration of key colleagues?

Having explicitly identified the barriers to implementation, you must next enlist the help of key colleagues. Occasionally it may be possible to implement the guideline in your own clinical practice first, although this will limit the potential benefits to all patients. To implement a hospital-wide guideline the cooperation of other clinicians, managers and administrators will be needed. Others may also have become involved in guideline development or appraisal: these colleagues may be particularly useful allies.

Question 3   Can you meet the educational, administrative and economic conditions necessary for the guideline's implementation?

Whenever a guideline is implemented there is likely to be a disturbance in the status quo that some individuals are likely to resist. There is evidence to suggest that certain measures can be taken to improve the likelihood that a clinical guideline will be adopted.

A credible synthesis of the evidence by a respected body is an important aid to guideline implementation. Furthermore, if local 'role models' are already implementing the guideline successfully, it is more likely that others will follow suit. It is also more likely to be implemented if consistent and coherent information is given. Important problems may be resolved by further discussion, preferably individually. When extensive cooperation is not assured, it may be best to focus on a smaller, targeted group of clinicians for whom success is more likely in the first instance. Relative freedom from conflict with other hospital initiatives is also an obvious requirement. Patients and their representatives may also have a view on whether the guideline introduction is a positive move, and it is important to canvass their opinion.

In our example the guideline appears to have been devised with a particular environment in mind. If, however, your colleagues seem receptive to the general principles of the guideline but wish for further discussion, it may be possible to ask one of the contributors to the guideline to visit to discuss it in more detail. The guideline has a summary and a quick-reference guide. You believe you can implement it locally and that it is consistent with the ethos that drug therapy may, in some circumstances, be harmful in this group of people.

Conclusions

Having reviewed this guideline, you decide it is valid, important, and can be used in caring for your own patients. You emphasize that there is an important need to adapt the guideline to reflect the local provision of service. You undertake to do this, and to arrange to monitor the outcomes of applying the guideline in your hospital.

Guidelines worksheet

Are the recommendations in this guideline valid?

1. Were all important decision options and outcomes clearly specified?

2. Was the evidence relevant to each decision option identified, validated and combined in a sensible and explicit way?

3. Are the relative preferences that key stakeholders attach to the outcomes of decisions (including benefits, risks and costs) identified and explicitly considered?

4. Is the guideline resistant to clinically sensible variations in practice?

Is this valid guideline or strategy potentially useful?

Does this guideline offer an opportunity for significant improvement in the quality of healthcare practice?

- Is there a large variation in current practice?

- Does the guideline contain new evidence (or old evidence not yet acted upon) that could have an important impact on management?

- Would the guideline affect the management of so many people, or concern individuals at such high risk, or involve such high costs that even small changes in practice could have major impacts on health outcomes or resources (including opportunity costs)?

Should this guideline or strategy be applied in your practice?

1. What barriers exist to its
   implementation?

   • Can they be overcome?

2. Can you enlist the collaboration of key
   colleagues?

3. Can you meet the educational,
   administrative, and economic
   conditions that are likely to determine
   the success or failure of implementing
   the strategy?

   • Credible synthesis of the evidence by
   a respected body

   • Respected, influential local
   exemplars already implementing the
   strategy

   • Consistent information from all
   relevant sources

   • Opportunity for individual discussions
   about the strategy with an authority

   • User-friendly format for guidelines

   • Implementable within target group of
   clinicians (without the need for
   extensive outside collaboration)

   • Freedom from conflict with economic
   incentives, administrative incentives,
   patient expectations, and community
   expectations.

CLINICAL AUDIT

A clinical audit (or, in the USA, clinical utilization review) paper differs in some ways from those addressing clinical research issues such as diagnosis and treatment. Importantly, there is no requirement for a control group. An audit project studies healthcare activity by scrutinizing how existing practice meets certain standards (Naylor & Guyatt 1996). Thus, audit is a pragmatic way of evaluating healthcare practices. The outcome of a particular practice depends on several factors, e.g. the severity of patients' illnesses, clinicians' preferences, etc. Even with the best evidence from research studies one would still be uncertain whether a particular healthcare activity is carried out appropriately and what outcome it produces in everyday clinical use. An audit can therefore determine what happens in actual practice, and to what effect.

Another distinctive feature of audit is the 'audit cycle'. As shown in Figure 4.4, this succinctly sets out the scope, purpose and anatomy of the audit process. As a process, the cycle refers to the fact that a successful audit will correct any deficit between actual practice and the standards set, i.e. audit is not simply monitoring, and 'closing the audit loop' is an important part.

Clinical scenario

You are posted to an ECT clinic for a week to train in specific skills for ECT administration. A journalist friend is horrified and shows you articles from popular daily newspapers which claim that psychiatrists use ECT irresponsibly. You ask your ECT consultant who gives you the following paper (Duffett & Lelliott 1998).

Précis of published article

Thirty-three ECT clinics in north east Thames and East Anglia and 17 clinics in Wales were visited for the evaluation of ECT practices using standards derived from the Royal College of Psychiatrists' ECT handbook (1995). Another 165 consultants with responsibility for ECT clinics in England were sent questionnaires to assess ECT practices, and 129 responded. These questionnaires were also completed by 10 of the consultants whose units were visited, to compare any inherent differences between the two methods. The areas of practice addressed were facilities, equipment, practice, personnel and training. In the clinics visited,

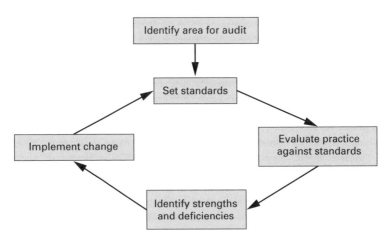

Fig. 4.8 The audit cycle

only 16% of the ECT consultants attended weekly and only 6% had sessions allocated to ECT. About 59% of clinics had machines recommended by the Royal College of Psychiatrists. Only one-third had clear policies to guide the junior doctors in administering ECT effectively. Other results are quoted later in this section.

Is the study valid?

Question 1 Did the audit use valid criteria or standards?

To perform an audit one should have set criteria against which practice can be evaluated. These should preferably be clinical guidelines based on a systematic review of all the available evidence. Local guidelines and even consensus statements may, however, be acceptable alternatives if they are the best evidence available. If there are no existing guidelines they could be drawn up following the procedure for developing clinical guidelines for good practice (see previous section).

You quickly read through the paper and find out that the standards selected are the Royal College of Psychiatrists' revised guidelines on the use of ECT.

Question 2 Was an explicit method used to identify and select the criteria/standard?

As with other evidence-based processes, the original standards should specify explicit criteria for identifying research papers that make up the guidelines. Inclusion and exclusion criteria should be specified at the outset of the paper selection process. This confirms that the guidelines were developed through a process of objective evidence seeking, rather than the mere consensus of 'experts'. Once research papers are selected, the methods used to synthesize and interpret data should be clearly stated.

The guideline does not specify the strategy used to identify research papers. It appears to be a collection of expert opinions. Although various experts have quoted various papers, a systematic literature search was not done to identify relevant papers.

Question 3 What is the quality of evidence used to frame the criteria?

One needs to know what sort of studies were used to design the guidelines. In a therapeutic situation, randomized controlled trials and meta-analyses would be particularly relevant evidence. Observational data and even consensus opinion could be used to fill up information lacunae. If this is the best available evidence, it is acceptable. This must, however, be clearly stated as the use of consensus opinion, even from 'experts', reduces the strength of the guideline.

Unfortunately, the guidelines do not specify any search strategy or study inclusion criteria in their preparation.

Question 4 How was expert opinion used in generating the criteria?

Expert opinion is unavoidable if data are lacking. In such cases, to increase the representativeness of collective opinion, the panel of experts should ideally be recruited from a variety of backgrounds. If the experts rated research papers to develop guidelines, it would be important to know whether and what objective criteria were used to do so, and how any disagreements in rating the research data were resolved (e.g. through a vote).

These details are not included in the published guidelines.

Question 5 How reliably were the criteria applied?

It is important to know how the criteria were actually used to assess current practice. This could involve formulating the guidelines into an objective schedule or scale to measure the activity being audited. Again, however, these details are not explicit in the Royal College of Psychiatrists' guidelines.

Question 6   Were the assessments prospective or retrospective?

Ideally all data collection should be prospective. Retrospective data collection is prone to recall bias, faulty or inconsistent reporting and incompleteness of data. Prospective assessments can be tailored to any kind of audit whether it is an assessment of facilities, activity or outcomes. Prospective data are, in short, more reliable.

The RCP audit uses a prospective approach to assess the ECT sites. The clinics were evaluated either by visits or by sending questionnaires to the ECT consultants.

Question 7   Were the criteria objective or subjective?

Several routine audits are performed using absolutely no objective criteria. No doubt readers will have experienced hospital audits where the assessments are done in a rather arbitrary manner, dependent upon the subjective impressions of the auditors. These are difficult to collate and analyse to make accurate generalizations. The particular healthcare activity needs to be broken down into components which can be assessed objectively. A checklist or questionnaire should be devised to assess these components. Ratings may involve the assignment of grades or descriptive terms. Each of these should be defined in a operational and objective manner. Finally, interrater reliability could be used to determine whether objective criteria were indeed developed and used appropriately.

The ECT audit assessments were done by using a schedule derived from the RCP handbook. This schedule and rating is not described in detail in the audit paper. Some scores involved 'yes' or 'no' responses, e.g. supervision of trainees giving ECT. However, there were items that used global impressions and ratings, such as 'good' or 'poor'. The paper does not mention whether operational criteria were used to qualify such impressions. Only one rater assessed all the sites, which is a source of potential subjective bias in rating even if objective criteria were used. The authors also sent a postal questionnaire to ECT consultants in sites that were not visited.

The development and any other quality of this questionnaire is not described. The authors conclude on the basis of 10 sites that were assessed by both methods, i.e. visit and postal questionnaire, that the results were 'sufficiently similar'. In the absence of any reliability statistic this statement has to be treated sceptically.

Are the results important?

Audit criteria may be based on sound evidence but be applied incorrectly. Therefore, before deciding whether an audit is useful in your setting, you must be satisfied that the criteria were applied correctly.

Question 1   Was the process of applying the criteria reliable, unbiased, and likely to lead to robust conclusions?

As already stated, it is not clear from the report whether the ratings were applied in a consistent fashion. This could lead to bias of various types and with various effects.

Fifty sites were visited and assessed. Questionnaires were sent to the rest and 129 (78%) of the 165 ECT consultants replied; 25% of the visited ECT suites were rated poor and 25% good. The comparable figures through questionnaires are 7% and 36%. These comparisons suggest that the auditors tended to rate the clinics lower than did the responsible consultants. In general, therefore, the overall results probably give an overoptimistic impression, as they mainly come from self-report questionnaire responses.

The overall performance of the clinics was better if the consultant had attended the ECT course organized by the college (7% versus 2%, $P<0.05$). These results suggest that attendance on the course was associated with better treatment, but this result could be confounded by doctors running better services being more likely to attend a course, i.e. cause and effect is difficult to establish here (as with all cross-sectional surveys).

Can I generalize the results to my setting?

Question 1   What sort of setting was studied in the audit?

The outcome of a healthcare practice may vary with the kind of setting, e.g. primary or tertiary care, teaching or district hospital, etc. You need to know whether the audit was carried out in centres similar to yours, or where ECT practice is similar to yours. This audit was carried out in ECT facilities in England and Wales. If your clinic is in this region or a similar one (e.g. Scotland) then the audit results are likely to be applicable.

Question 2   How extensive was the audit and how were the samples selected?

It is obvious that an audit should cover as many clinical settings and services as possible, and that they are representative of all settings and services. Biases may otherwise be introduced, e.g. through the auditors' inability to visit all the sites, or even a representative sample, because of distances involved or lack of manpower. With respect to self-report questionnaires, there may be bias due to non-response or to socially desirable responses.

The audit covered several hospitals in England and Wales, but the authors do not make it clear how centres for the visit were selected. Only two regions of England were visited, the rest of the centres being evaluated by questionnaires sent to the consultants. The response rate of these questionnaires was reasonable (78%). Therefore, the results from questionnaires, assuming a degree of reliability, may be more indicative of national practices. The authors quote that a small sample who were both administered questionnaire and had visits scored 'similar' on both the ratings. This may be so, but clearly the results show that some outcomes were markedly different, e.g. the quality ratings of the ECT suite were markedly better in self-report questionnaires than with actual site visits. The authors report data pooled from the questionnaires and site visits, which makes it difficult to be sure that the findings apply to your setting.

There could be other potential sources of bias, e.g. if the visited clinics were informed in advance about the visit. Ideally, surprise visits should be made to assess true practice quality, as there maybe a tendency to adhere more strictly to guidelines if the centre is prepared, but obviously this may be impractical. The authors of the audit do not state whether the visited sites were informed in advance or not.

Question 3   Have the criteria been field tested?

A field-tested guideline is likely to have more validity and generalizability than one just drawn up on paper. It is, for example, important to know whether any treatment studies are practical and if there are any important omissions. This criterion may, however, be difficult to meet, as it would require 'closing the loop' by reaudit.

The RCP guidelines have been field tested and updated. This is the third edition. There is clearly still scope for the improvement of ECT facilities and treatments, but this requires time and money.

Conclusions

The methodological limitations of the paper have been discussed but it still yields valuable information in the absence of any other similar audit. The results are likely to apply to your setting. It is clear that ECT practice varies across the country, but this does not mean it is irresponsible. You attempt to discuss the results and their implications with your journalist friend who is somewhat reassured but does not think the audit is newsworthy.

Worksheets

Is the audit valid?

1. Was an explicit and sensible process used to identify, select and combine evidence for the criteria?

2. What is the quality of the evidence used in framing the criteria?

3. Where expert opinion was used, was an explicit, systematic and reliable process used?

4. Was an explicit and sensible process used to consider the relative values of different outcomes?

5. If the quality of the evidence is weak, have the criteria been correlated with patient outcomes?

Are the results important?

1. Was the process for applying the criteria reliable, unbiased and likely to yield robust conclusions?

2. What is the impact of uncertainty associated with evidence and values on the criteria-based ratings of process of care?

Can I use this audit study in caring for my patient(s)?

---

1. Are the criteria relevant to my practice
   setting?

---

2. How similar is the audit study to your
   own clinical practice?

---

3. Have the criteria been field tested?

REFERENCES AND FURTHER READING

Altman DG, Anderson PK 1999 Calculating the number needed to treat for trials
where the outcome is time to an event. British Medical Journal 319: 1492–1495

Arnold VK, Rosenthal, TL, Dupont, RT, Hilliard D 1993 Redundant clothing: a readily
observable marker for schizophrenia in the psychiatric emergency room
population. Journal of Behavioural Therapeutic and Experimental Psychiatry 24:
45–47

Briggs A 1999 Economics notes. Handling uncertainty in economic evaluation.
British Medical Journal 319: 120

Buchanan A 1998 Criminal conviction after discharge from special (high security)
hospital: incidence in the first 10 years. British Journal of Psychiatry 172:
472–476

Drummond MF, Stoddart GL, Torrance W 1997a Methods for the economic
evaluation of healthcare programmes, 2nd edn. Oxford: Oxford University Press

Drummond MF, Richardson WS, O'Brien BJ, Levine M, Heyland D 1997b Users' guides
to the medical literature. XIII. How to use an article on economic analysis of clinical
practice. A. Are the results of the study valid? The Evidence-Based Medicine
Working Group. Journal of the American Medical Association 277: 1552–1557

Duffett R, Lelliott P 1998 Auditing electroconvulsive therapy. The third cycle. British
Journal of Psychiatry 172: 401–405

Glennie JL 1997 Pharmacoeconomic evaluations of clozapine in treatment-resistant
schizophrenia and risperidone in chronic schizophrenia. 7. The Canadian
coordinating office for health technology assessment. Technology overview: URL:
www.ccohta.ca

Guyatt GH, Sackett DL, Cook DJ 1993 Users' guides to the medical literature: II.
How to use an article about therapy or prevention: A. Are the results of the study
valid? Journal of the American Medical Association 270: 2598–2601

Guyatt GH, Sackett DL, Cook DJ 1994 Users' guides to the medical literature: II. How to use an article about therapy or prevention: B. What were the results and will they help me in caring for my patients? Journal of the American Medical Association 271: 59–63

Hayward RS, Wilson MC, Tunis SR, Bass EB, Guyatt G 1995 Users' guides to the medical literature. VIII. How to use clinical practice guidelines. A. Are the recommendations valid? The Evidence-Based Medicine Working Group. Journal of the American Medical Association 274: 570–574

Jacobson SJ, Jones K, Johnson K et al 1992 Prospective multicentre study of pregnancy outcome after lithium exposure during first trimester. Lancet 339: 530–533

Jefferson T, Demicheli V, Mugford M 1996 Elementary economic evaluation in healthcare. London: BMJ Publishing Group

Kennedy E, Song F, Hunter R, Clark A, Gilbody S 1999 Risperidone versus typical antipsychotic medication for schizophrenia. In: The Cochrane Library, Issue 4. Update Software

Laupacis A, Wells G, Richardson WS, Tugwell P 1994 Users' guides to the medical literature. V. How to use an article about prognosis. The Evidence-Based Medicine Working Group. Journal of the American Medical Association 272: 234–237

Levine M, Walter S, Lee H, Holbrook A, Moyer V 1994 Users' guides to the medical literature: IV. How to use an article about harm. Journal of the American Medical Association 271: 1615–1619

Naylor CD, Guyatt GH 1996 Users' guides to the medical literature. XI. How to use an article about a clinical utilization review. The Evidence-Based Medicine Working Group. Journal of the American Medical Association 275: 1435–1439

O'Brien BJ, Heyland D, Richardson WS, Levine M, Drummond MF 1997 Users' guides to the medical literature. XIII. How to use an article on economic analysis of clinical practice. B. What are the results and will they help me in caring for my patients? The Evidence-Based Medicine Working Group. Journal of the American Medical Association 277: 1802–1806

Oxman AD, Cook DJ, Guyatt GH 1994 Users' guides to the medical literature: VI. How to use an overview. Journal of the American Medical Association 272: 1367–1371

Roman J, Guyatt GH, Sackett DL 1994a Users' guides to the medical literature: III. how to use an article about a diagnostic test: A. Are the results of the study valid? Journal of the American Medical Association 271: 389–391

Roman J, Guyatt GH, Sackett DL 1994b Users' guides to the medical literature: III. How to use an article about a diagnostic test: B. What are the results and will they help me in caring for my patients? Journal of the American Medical Association 271: 703–707

Royal College of Psychiatrists 1995 The ECT handbook: 2nd report of the Royal College of Phsyciatrists Special Committee on ECT. Council Reports CR39. Royal College of Psychiatrists, London

Sackett DL, Straus SE, Richardson WS, Rosenberg W, Haynes RB 2000 Evidence-based medicine, 2nd editon. Churchill Livingstone, Edinburgh

Scottish Intercollegiate Guidelines Network (SIGN) 1998 Interventions in the management of behavioural and psychological aspects of dementia. Pilot. Edinburgh: Scottish Intercollegiate Guidelines Network

Tarrier N, Yusupoff L, Kinney C et al 1998 Randomized controlled trial of intensive cognitive behaviour therapy for patients with chronic schizophrenia. British Medical Journal 317: 303–307

Wilson MC, Hayward RS, Tunis SR, Bass EB, Guyatt G 1995 Users' guides to the Medical Literature. VIII. How to use clinical practice guidelines. B. what are the recommendations and will they help you in caring for your patients? The Evidence-Based Medicine Working Group. Journal of the American Medical Association 274: 1630–1632

REVISION MCQs

Q1 The number needed to treat (NNT):

(a) Is the reciprocal of the relative risk reduction
(b) For time to an event should be carefully specified with regard to the duration of the study
(c) Is the same as the effect size statistic
(d) May have confidence intervals that cross infinity if a statistically insignificant result is found
(e) Is defined as the number of people needed to treat with a new rather than a control treatment to prevent one outcome

Q2 In appraising treatment studies:

(a) The NNT is the most important consideration
(b) Patient values and preferences are important
(c) An effect size statistic may be calculated for studies that employ continuous outcome measures
(d) Confidence intervals should be used to measure the precision of an NNT
(e) An attrition rate of more than 30% may seriously jeopardize the conclusions of a treatment study

Q3 A sensitivity analysis:

(a) May be conducted using a 'Monte Carlo' analysis

(b) May be based on stochastic methods

(c) Is a technique specific to economic analyses

(d) When the conclusions of an economic study hold for a very rigorous sensitivity analysis, the reader may have more confidence in its conclusion

(e) Can not be applied to a cost-effectiveness analysis

Q4 The following statements are true:

(a) Cost–benefit analysis is much more common than cost-effectiveness analysis in the health economics field

(b) Economically, treatments should be purchased if they are more effective than existing treatment, regardless of the cost

(c) A treatment is cost-effective if the cost per unit health gain is lower than a control treatment

(d) Incremental costs are sometimes used to indicate the cost required to bring about one additional beneficial outcome

(e) The validity of an economic analysis, based on a meta-analysis, does not depend on the validity of the meta-analysis

Q5 The validity of a guideline depends upon:

(a) The degree of variation in current clinical practice

(b) Opportunity costs

(c) Whether patients and their representatives were consulted during its development

(d) Complete agreement between all of the relevant stakeholders

(e) A non-systematic review of the literature

Q6 Evidence-based guidelines:

(a) May be based on clinical consensus alone

(b) If produced by a 'clinical expert' need not use stringent methodology

(c) Are useful when key collaborators can be enlisted

(d) Cannot be applied to diagnostic investigations

(e) Can be sufficiently stated as a flow diagram

Q7 Diagnostic studies:

(a) Should compare a diagnostic test with a 'gold standard'

(b) Measure the concurrent validity of a diagnostic test

(c) With a high specificity suggest that a negative test rules out the disorder

(d) A sensitive test identifies a high proportion of people with the target disorder

(e) The receiver operator characteristic may be a useful aid to deciding a diagnostic threshold

Q8 The following statements about the appraisal of diagnostic studies are true:

(a) The post-test odds for a positive test are the odds of someone with a positive test having the disorder

(b) The likelihood ratio for a positive test is the post-test odds divided by the pretest odds

(c) The likelihood ratio for a positive result after two positive and separate diagnostic tests can be estimated by multiplying the likelihood ratios together

(d) The positive predictive value is unrelated to the disease prevalence

(e) Sensitivity and specificity are independent

Q9 The following considerations are important in evaluating the validity of a meta-analysis:

(a) The sources of the included studies

(b) If a systematic review was conducted

. (c) If any attempt was made to deal with publication bias

(d) Some measure of methodological rigour of the original studies was specified

(e) Heterogeneity

Q10 Prognostic factors are:

(a) The same as risk factors

(b) Studied using a cohort design

(c) Causal factors in a given condition

(d) Quantified using odds ratios

(e) Decided by clinical consensus

Q11 The following can confound a prognosis study:

(a) Varying patient ages

(b) Different points in the illness course
(c) Several raters
(d) Use of non-parametric statistics
(e) Subjective assessment of outcome

Q12 The following issues can be answered reliably by a cohort study:

(a) Treatment efficacy
(b) Disease course
(c) Disease biology
(d) Incidence of the disease
(e) Survival statistics

ANSWERS

A1

(a) False (the absolute risk reduction)
(b) True
(c) False (this is used for continuous measures)
(d) True (if the CI of the ARR includes zero)
(e) True

A2

(a) False (validity and applicability are at least as important)
(b) True
(c) True
(d) True
(e) True

A3

(a) True
(b) True (variables with a mean and variance)
(c) False (also used in meta-analyses and diagnoses)
(d) True
(e) False

A4

(a) False (generally the reverse is the case)

(b) False
(c) True
(d) True
(e) False (the validity of the study is important)

A5

(a) False (this relates to usefulness)
(b) True (whether there are other interventions where resources could be allocated)
(c) True
(d) False (not necessary, but disagreement should be explicitly stated)
(e) False (guidelines must undertake a systematic review)

A6

(a) False (these would be consensus guidelines)
(b) False
(c) True
(d) False
(e) False (this is not sufficient)

A7

(a) True
(b) True (another term for a comparison with an accepted 'gold standard')
(c) False (a positive test rules in the disorder – SpIn)
(d) True
(e) True (the 'knee' or 'shoulder' may be used when sensitivity and specificity are equally important)

A8

(a) True
(b) True
(c) True
(d) False (this rises with disease prevalence)
(e) False (sensitivity falls as specificity rises and vice versa)

A9

(a) True
(b) True
(c) True (by contacting pharmaceutical companies, funnel plots, etc.)
(d) True
(e) True (the degree to which the results of included studies vary more than expected by chance alone)

A10

(a) False
(b) True
(c) False (associated, not necessarily causal)
(d) True (although relative risks are arguably more useful)
(e) False

A11

(a) True
(b) True
(c) False (this is not strictly a confounder)
(d) False (this is a statistical issue)
(e) False (this is bias, not confounding)

A12

(a) True (the RCT is a specific form of cohort study)
(b) True
(c) True
(d) True (an unaffected cohort needs to be studied)
(e) True

Mock exam papers and model answers

The following mock exam papers are based on the format of the critical appraisal paper for the MRCPsych part II. In each case we give a short account of a piece of research, followed by questions and brief model answers, with total marks of 100. These are of course likely to be particularly useful for trainees about to sit the exam, both as exam practice and to identify any topics that require more attention, but they could also be used by any reader to assess their understanding and knowledge. We have obviously identified the topic of an article/exam by the subheadings, which will not be the case in the exam, but this is rarely a major source of difficulty and will help you identify your strengths and weaknesses. We have generally based our questions on a published paper and refer to this at the start of each section. You may find it useful to obtain the article – after you have attempted the exam – as the discussion sections in particular may shed further light on why a question was asked, or on our model answer. Note, however, that inclusion in this chapter does not imply that we think the article is necessarily a valid piece of scientific research.

At the time of writing there have only been two formal exams and two example papers circulated by the College. The pilot paper was in two sections, marked out of 150, and lasted 1 hour. A sample paper circulated by the College was in one section, allotted 45 minutes and marked out of 110. Both of these and a number of other mock exam papers are published by Brown & Wilkinson (1998), a second edition of which will be available shortly. The first and second actual exam papers were in two sections, to be answered over 90 minutes and given 100 marks in total (70 and 30 respectively, with 10 marks for each question). The latter format is obviously the best guide to future exams, but it may change. We have decided to allocate 45 minutes to our mock exam papers and mark them out of 100 for convenience, as we are writing more than revision text, but you could attempt two questions in 90 minutes as a more formal mock exam if you wish.

These short examples should be approached as one would prepare for the exam proper. You might find it useful to read through the questions first to help you focus on the most relevant parts of the text. Do not be surprised if later questions in the paper help you answer one or two of the earlier questions. Short answers with key pieces of information are sufficient for most answers, as the exam is probably marked according to mention or not of such key phrases – we have used brief sentences and a simple scoring scheme to facilitate marking. Above all, try to ensure that you attempt each and every question – there is no negative marking and anything (even a wild guess) is more likely to get you some marks than nothing. We think, however, that it is possible to get 100% in this part of the exam, particularly if you have read this book right through.

Good luck.

DIAGNOSIS I

Read the following abridged paper carefully and then answer questions 1–6 at the end.

The paper studies the usefulness of a screening questionnaire in diagnosing depression, but is a made-up example for this mock exam, rather than being an account of previously published research.

Précis

This (mock) study aims to identify a reliable screening test for depression in primary care. Patients were approached at four large urban Edinburgh general practices. A trained researcher gave a brief standardized explanation of the study. Patients could either agree to participate, in which case they were asked to complete the questionnaire, or they were directed to the waiting room without a questionnaire. Questionnaires were retrieved by the GP but were not used as a source of clinical information. On leaving the consultation room subjects were seen by a second investigator, who administered the structured clinical interview for DSM-IV. No experimenter had access to the findings of the other and the clinical interview was applied regardless of the results of the test. The study was continued until 100 patients with a current DSM-IV diagnosis of major depression were recruited.

One hundred patients with a current DSM-IV diagnosis of major depression were recruited, along with 400 people without; 30 patients with other psychiatric illnesses were included in both groups. These were classified as cases if the DSM-IV criteria for MDD (major depressive disorder) were met, and as non-cases free from MDD if the criteria were not met.

Four cut-offs were examined. Of the 15 questions, cut-offs of 6, 8, 10 and 12 were used to define caseness, and their sensitivity and specificity calculated. The results are given in Table 5.1.

Table 5.1   The performance of the diagnostic test at different cut-offs

Cut-off	Sensitivity	Specificity	1 – specificity
6	0.995	0.4	0.6
8	0.89	0.6	0.4
10	0.68	0.84	0.16
12	0.3	0.97	0.03

The results of the table are shown in Figure 5.1.

Questions

1. Describe (briefly) the three main reasons why this study is a valid measure of the screening test? (15 marks)

2. Define the likelihood ratio for a positive test. (10 marks)

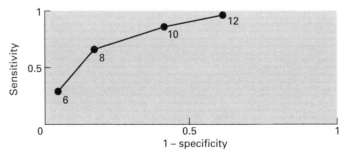

Fig. 5.1   Sensitivity and 1 – specificity at the four cut-offs.

3. What is the likelihood ratio for a positive test at each cut-off?
(15 marks)

4. Which cut-off would you use in your general practice, where the prevalence of depression is 1 in 6 of your outpatients? What would the test's positive predictive value be at your chosen cut-off? (25 marks)

5. What is the relationship between sensitivity and specificity? What factors should be considered when choosing a sensitive but non-specific test over a non-specific but highly sensitive test? (20 marks)

6. You decide to use six positive answers as your cut-off in a sample of patients of whom 10% have depression. You also employ a second test whose likelihood ratio is 12. What would be the probability of someone having depression if they were positive for both tests? (15 marks)

Answers

1. The diagnostic test was compared with a 'gold standard' by a separate investigator (5 marks). It is likely that this means they were not aware of the results of the first investigator (5 marks), although this is not stated conclusively in the text. The diagnostic test seems to have been compared with the 'gold standard' irrespective of the result (5 marks).

2. The likelihood ratio for a positive test is the value that test result has in predicting the presence of the target disorder (5 marks). It is the ratio of the proportion of positive test results in people with the disorder to the proportion of positive tests in those without the disorder (5 marks). (See Chapter 4 for details.)

3. The likelihood ratio for a positive test at each cut-off is LR = sens/(1 – spec). Therefore, LR+(6) = 1.66, LR+(8) = 2.23, LR+(10) = 4.25, LR+(12) = 10. (3 marks for each correct answer, 15 marks only if all four correct.)

4. If the prevalence of depression were 15% in your outpatients, what cut-off would you use?

Prevalence = 1/6, pretest odds = 1/6th/(1 – 1/6th) = 1/5 = 0.2 (5 marks).

Therefore, for each cut-off what would be the post-test probability for a positive result (i.e. the PPV), and a negative result (i.e. 1 – NPV)?

(Method: Post-test odds = pretest odds × LR. Then convert post-test odds back to probabilities using $P = O/(1 + O)$ (5 marks)

Cut-off	LR+	LR–	PPV	1 – NPV	NPV
6	1.66	0.0125	0.249	0.0025	0.9975
8	2.23	0.183	0.308	0.0353	0.9647
10	4.25	0.381	0.459	0.0708	0.93
12	10	0.722	0.667	0.126	0.874

Given that the prevalence of depression in your practice is 1/6, the PPV will be lower than that of the study (where the prevalence was 20%) and the NPV will be higher. A cut-off of 10 would mean only 45.9% (calculated from post-TO = LR+ × pre-TO) of those positive for the test would actually have depression (5 marks). This would probably incur a vastly increased workload for the GP and needless extra investigation (5 marks). Therefore, a cut-off of 12 would probably be more satisfactory, as a higher proportion (66.7%) of those with a positive test would be true positives (5 marks).

5. Sensitivity generally increases as specificity falls for a diagnostic test, and vice versa (5 marks). Sensitive tests should be used where it is important to identify all possible cases of illness and miss very few (SnOut). Such a situation might arise where the consequences of missing a highly treatable disorder are very great (5 marks). A specific test is used where it is important that the majority of positive test results do indeed indicate the presence of the target disorder (SpIn) (5 marks). Such a situation may arise when a positive test would involve intensive, expensive and unpleasant investigation or treatment, or where the consequences of missing affected individuals is low and effective therapy is lacking (5 marks).

6. For 6+ answers the LR = 1.66. The new test LR = 12. Therefore the likelihood ratio for a positive result on both tests is 12 × 1.66 = 20 (approx.) (5 marks). If pre-test probability = 10%, pre-test odds = 1/9. Therefore:

Post-test odds = $1/9 \times 20 = 2.22$ (5 marks)

Post-test probability = $2.22/3.22 = 0.689$

Therefore, there is a 68.9% chance that someone positive for both tests would actually have the disorder (5 marks).

DIAGNOSIS II

The following information is taken from a paper on a new screening test for eating disorders (Morgan et al 1999). Read the text carefully and answer the questions at the end of the paper.

Précis

The researchers developed five questions addressing core features of anorexia nervosa and bulimia nervosa using focus groups of patients with eating disorders and specialists in eating disorders. The 'SCOFF' questionnaire (see Box 5.1) was tested in a feasibility study of patients and staff at an eating disorders unit. None of these participants was involved in the subsequent study.

They recruited cases sequentially from referrals to a specialist clinic: 116 women aged 18–40 years who were confirmed as having either anorexia nervosa ($n = 68$) or bulimia ($n = 48$), according to the criteria specified in the *Diagnostic and statistical manual of mental disorders*, fourth edition. They also recruited 96 women aged 18–39, through advertising by local colleges, who were confirmed as not having an eating disorder. Cases and controls were asked the SCOFF questions orally; they also completed the eating disorders inventory and the BITE self-rating scale for bulimia.

More cases than controls were in higher socioeconomic groups ($P<0.01$, $\chi^2 = 47.4$, df = 3) and cases were more likely to be single,

---

Box 5.1   The SCOFF questionnaire*

Do you make yourself **S**ick because you feel uncomfortably full?
Do you worry you have lost **C**ontrol over how much you eat?
Have you recently lost more than **O**ne stone in a 3-month period?
Do you believe yourself to be **F**at when others say you are too thin?
Would you say **F**ood dominates your life?

*One point for every 'yes'.

separated or divorced ($P<0.001$, $\chi^2 = 13.0$, df = 1). Mean length
of illness was 8 years. All scores on the eating disorders inventory
and the BITE scale were consistent with published data for women
with or without eating disorders. Specificity and sensitivity data for
the various cut-offs are given in Table 5.2 and a ROC curve is
shown in Figure 5.2.

Table 5.2   The sensitivity, specificity, positive predictive value and negative
predictive value of SCOFF questionnaire for all cases versus all controls

Cut-off	Sensitivity	PPV	Specificity	NPV
2	100	90.6	87.5	100
3	99.1	96.6	95.8	98.9
4	87.9	100	100	93.2

Questions

1. Do you think this study uses valid methodology?   (20 marks)

2. There were differences between cases and controls at the start
   of the study. What effect might this have had on the results
   obtained?   (10 marks)

3. What are the pretest odds of eating disorders in this sample?
   (10 marks)

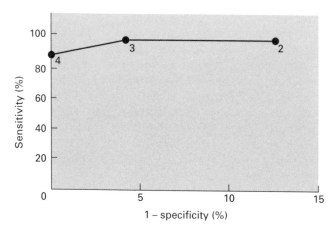

Fig. 5.2   ROC curve of sensitivity versus 1 – specificity at various cut-offs
on the SCOFF questionnaire.

4. What unusual characteristic does the LR- at a cut-off of 2 have? What does this mean? (10 marks)

5. The test in the study was administered to people from an eating disorders service compared with those from local colleges. How might the test have behaved if it had been administered to consecutive patients from a psychiatric outpatient clinic with the same prevalence of eating disorders? (10 marks)

6. What clinical and mathematical factors should you consider when deciding what cut-off to choose on a diagnostic test? How do you decide which cut-off to choose? (20 marks)

7. What is a ROC curve, why is it used and how does it help you decide on specific diagnostic thresholds? (20 marks)

Answers

1. We are told that all cases and controls completed the SCOFF questionnaire regardless of the test result (5 marks). However, it is not clear whether investigators did this blind to the results of the other test or not (5 marks). The test was validated on samples from an eating disorder clinic (cases) and local colleges (controls), i.e. different populations (5 marks). This possible non-blinding and non-independence is a limitation of the study, but is probably not sufficient to invalidate its findings (5 marks).

2. There were significant differences in social class and marital status between cases and controls. Cases were more likely to be single, separated or divorced and in higher socioeconomic classes. The former could be attributable to the illness, but the latter is likely to represent bias. Patients who volunteer for studies such as this may not be representative of patients (with eating disorders) as a whole. The difference between cases and controls may illustrate this. Therefore, the results in clinical practice may differ systematically from the behaviour of this test in a research context (10 marks).

3. There were 116 cases and 96 controls. Therefore, the prevalence of eating disorders in this sample is 116/212 = 54.7% (5 marks). The pretest odds were therefore 116/96 = 1.21 (5 marks).

4. The likelihood ratio (negative test) at a cut-off of 2 is 0 (5 marks). This means that the value of a negative result in predicting the presence of the disorder is 0, or that a negative test is infinitely more likely to come from someone without the disorder than someone with (10 marks).

5. If the test had been administered to a patient sample, its ability to distinguish between those with the disorder and those with a common differential diagnosis (e.g. depressive disorder) is likely to be reduced (5 marks). Therefore, specificity and the positive predictive value may reduce. Sensitivity and the negative predictive value are less likely to be reduced, as the test would still be able to identify those with the disorder to the same extent, but would probably include extra cases of people without the disorder. To answer this question definitively, the study should be repeated on just such a sample. (5 marks for a discussion of how any two of sensitivity, specificity, PPV or NPV might change.)

6. Factors to consider when choosing a cut-off are:

   Mathematically: The sensitivity (ability to rule out)
   The specificity (ability to rule in)
   The PPV (the 'true positive' rate)
   The NPV (the 'true negative' rate)
   (Any 2 = 10 marks)

   Clinically: The costs and consequences of untreated illness
   The availability and effectiveness of treatment
   The unpleasantness of further investigation and treatment   (Any 2 = 10 marks)

7. The ROC curve relates sensitivity to 1 − specificity at different diagnostic thresholds (5 marks). It was originally used by air traffic controllers. It can be used to effectively choose the cut-off that optimizes both the sensitivity and specificity of a test (5 marks) by choosing the knee (or shoulder) of the ROC curve (5 marks) or by choosing the diagnostic test that maximizes the area under the curve when more than one test is available (5 marks).

Acknowledgements
We wish to thank the authors of this paper for allowing us access to their data.

TREATMENT I

Read the following abridged paper (Elliot et al 1998) carefully and then answer questions 1–10 at the end.

Précis

There were 132 HIV-positive persons screened for entry to the study. Of these, 57 were excluded because of poor compliance ($n = 20$), bipolar disorder ($n = 8$), substance misuse ($n = 12$), current antidepressant treatment ($n = 9$), failure to meet diagnostic criteria ($n = 5$) and severe medical illness ($n = 3$). Therefore, 75 subjects were included in the trial. They had a mean age of 36 years (SD = 7.5).

Subjects were randomly assigned to blind treatment with placebo ($n = 25$), imipramine ($n = 25$) or paroxetine ($n = 25$). Paroxetine was increased to 40 mg from 20 mg if tolerated. Imipramine was started at 50 mg and increased to 100 mg or 200 mg over 3 weeks if tolerated. Assessments were made at baseline and weeks 2, 4, 6, 8 and 12. Subject who did not show a response at 6 weeks, as measured by a 25% reduction in the Hamilton Depression Rating Scale, were withdrawn because of ethical concerns.

Current diagnoses were assessed using the structured clinical interview for DSM-III-R (SCID). Subjects with a diagnosis of major depression and a score of 18 or more on the Hamilton Depression Rating Scale (HDRS) entered the trial. Subjects were repeatedly assessed using the HDRS and the clinical global impression (CGI) scale and the brief symptom inventory. CD4 cell counts were also made at weeks 0 and 12, along with AIDS-defining symptoms, to rate individuals according to CDC criteria: asymptomatic HIV, symptomatic HIV and AIDS.

Continuous data were analysed by means of a one-way analysis of variance (ANOVA) and by the χ^2 test for categorical data. Response to medication was examined using repeated measures ANOVA of the HDRS at each assessment and the CGI scale. The data were analysed using intention-to-treat analysis for part of the study, and last observation carried forward for those patients who completed 4 weeks of the trial.

Using the χ^2 statistic the proportion of responders in each group was analysed. Partial response was a reduction of 50% in the HDRS from baseline to week 12; a full response was defined as an

HDRS score of less than 8. For the CGI a response was defined as a score of 1 or 2 on the scale.

There were no significant differences between the groups in terms of the participant characteristics. Active treatment for at least 6 weeks was received by 56 (75%) of the 75 subjects, and 34 (45%) of the subjects completed the entire 12-week trial (placebo $n = 13$, paroxetine $n = 11$, imipramine $n = 10$). All paroxetine-treated patients received at least 20 mg/day; 44% of the intention-to-treat imipramine-treated group completed the trial using at least 150 mg of imipramine per day.

Analysis of the response of subjects who completed the trial showed significant effects on HDRS scores for drug and time, and also on CGI score for the drug. Post-hoc analysis revealed less consistent effects. Only imipramine was superior to placebo at week 12 ($F = 4.29$, df = 2,31, $P<0.05$) for HDRS and CGI score.

The results from the intention-to-treat analysis are given in Table 5.3.

Table 5.3 Intention-to-treat analysis. Results at week 12: numbers of people showing a response to medication

Measure	Placebo		Paroxetine		Imipramine		Analysis	
	n	%	n	%	n	%	χ^2 (df = 2)	Imip vs parox
HDRS	9	40.9	9	50	13	81.3	6.41	NS
CGI	4	18.2	6	33.3	12	75	12.93	$P<0.05$

Questions

Please write your answers to questions 1–10 on a separate sheet.

1. Describe how exactly 25 patients could have been randomized to each group in the trial. What method can be used to ensure equal numbers? (10 marks)

2. Were the dropout rates in the three groups equal, and why is this important? (10 marks)

3. At week 6 subjects could be removed from the trial because of a lack of response. How could this have led to problems with the study and why? (5 marks)

4. What is an intention-to-treat analysis and why is it used? (10 marks)

5. In terms of the HDRS scores, what is the response rate for paroxetine-treated patients compared with that for imipramine-treated patients? What is the absolute risk reduction and the number needed to treat? (15 marks)

6. In terms of the CGI what is the response rate for paroxetine-treated patients compared with that for imipramine-treated patients? What are the absolute risk reduction and the number needed to treat? Why is this figure different from that calculated above? (15 marks)

7. Is clinical significance the same as statistical significance? Indicate in your answer what you understand by these terms. (10 marks)

8. You are asked by the local infectious disease unit to assess an inpatient who has AIDS. He is 28 years old and depressed, with 'biological symptoms'. Can this study be applied to this patient? (5 marks)

9. This single study reports an estimate of the treatment effect of imipramine and paroxetine compared with placebo. What prior calculation could the authors of this paper have performed to ensure there were enough subjects to detect a statistically significant difference? (10 marks)

10. You are not satisfied with the results of a single study and decide to look for a meta-analysis. What is a meta-analysis and what are its strengths and weaknesses compared with a single RCT? (10 marks)

Answers

1. Randomization could have been by blocks, where equal numbers are assured. For example, if A, B and C represent different treatment groups, randomization by the following blocks would ensure equal numbers in each group: ABC, ACB, BAC, BCA, CBA, CAB (10 marks).

2. The dropout rates were 12/25 (48%), 11/25 (56%) and 15/25 (60%), i.e. the numbers that dropped out in each group were approximately equal (5 marks). Unequal dropout rates can lead to biased results (5 marks).

3. At 6 weeks some subjects may have been removed who would subsequently have shown a response to treatment. In the intention-to-treat analysis of this study these subjects would have been considered treatment failures (5 marks).

4. An intention-to-treat analysis is where the patients' scores are analysed in the groups to which they were randomized (5 marks), i.e. all patients contribute to the results. The rationale for this is that dropouts generally do so because of adverse events or treatment failure, so that not including them in the analysis will overestimate the effect of a new drug treatment (5 marks).

5. For the HDRS the paroxetine response rate is 50% and the imipramine response rate is 81.3% (5 marks). The absolute risk reduction is 81.3%–50% = 31.3% (5 marks). Therefore, the number needed to treat is 4 (5 marks) (rounded up to the nearest integer).

6. For the CGI the paroxetine response rate is 33.3% and the imipramine response rate is 75%. The absolute risk reduction is 75%–33.3% = 41.7% (5 marks). Therefore, the number needed to treat is 3 (rounded up to the nearest integer) (5 marks). This figure is different from that from the HDRS as the CGI compares clinicians' ratings, whereas the HDRS compares an arbitrary cut-off on a rating scale. They are not directly comparable measures (5 marks).

7. Statistical significance is achieved when a result is unlikely to have occurred by chance alone. A 5% possibility that a result occurred by chance is usually taken as the arbitrary level of statistical significance (5 marks). Clinical significance refers to whether a treatment makes a sizeable contribution to a patient's wellbeing. A study may have a statistically significant result although the treatment does not alter a patient's wellbeing significantly (5 marks).

8. No. A 28-year-old inpatient may be unlike the people used in the study, who were an average age of 36, outpatients, and without severe medical illness (5 marks).

9. A power calculation could have been performed (5 marks). This is a technique used to estimate the sample size needed based on the estimated effect size or standardized difference expected and the statistical significance required (5 marks).

10. A meta-analysis is a mathematical combination of two or more studies weighted for quality and/or precision (5 marks). Its strengths include an increased power to detect treatment effects, potentially more precise estimates of treatment efficacy, and greater external validity if based on a wider range of patient characteristics. Its weaknesses include that it may be very misleading if unsystematic, may be subject to publication bias, is labour intensive, and may combine studies that are conducted in such disparate ways as to be incomparable (5 marks for any one advantage and disadvantage).

TREATMENT II

Read the following abridged paper (Klein et al 1999) carefully and then answer the six questions at the end of the paper.

Précis

Seventy-nine patients with DSM-IV major depressive disorder were invited to participate in a study of transcranial magnetic stimulation (TMS), of whom 70 gave written informed consent. The demographic and clinical characteristics are given in Table 5.4. Diagnosis was established by two senior psychiatrists following an extended clinical interview. All patients scored 15 or more on the Hamilton Depression Rating Scale (HDRS) and none was treatment resistant.

Table 5.4 Baseline characteristics of experimental and control groups

Variable	TMS ($n = 36$)	Sham TMS ($n = 34$)	Significance
Mean age (SD)	60.5 (15.1)	58.9 (18.3)	NS
Sex (F/M)	29/7	28/6	NS
Melancholia (y/n)	27/9	18/16	$P = 0.05$
History of MDD	29/7	20/14	$P < 0.05$
Other treatment	23/36	23/34	NS

Patients were maintained on their previous treatment regimen throughout the course of the study. None was receiving psychotherapy during the course of the study. Patients were randomly assigned to receive TMS or sham-TMS by a computer-generated random number list.

A magnetic stimulator (Cadwell Inc.) was used in the study. Initially motor thresholds were established over the right motor cortex by determining the minimum stimulus to produce a motor response in the left distal wrist muscles. During the treatment, the coil was placed over the right prefrontal area and a train of 60 stimuli was administered over 1 minute, followed by a 2-minute gap, and then another 1-minute train of 60 stimuli was administered.

During the sham treatment the coil was placed perpendicular to the scalp surface without direct contact, thereby minimizing the flow of energy into the skull. Stimulation parameters were otherwise the same.

Clinical ratings were assessed at baseline (before treatment), after five sessions (1 week), and 24 hours after the last session. The HDRS (17–item version) and the Montgomery–Asberg Depression Rating Scale (MADRS) were used to assess depressive symptoms and on a 7–point clinical global impression scale. The rater was a senior psychiatrist who was involved in the diagnostic evaluation but blind to the nature of treatment. In addition, the rater avoided asking questions that could disclose the nature of treatment.

Sixty-seven patients who initially started the study completed the entire protocol. The other three withdrew after five sessions for clinical reasons.

A clear difference was noted between the two groups after week 1, which continued throughout the study. The TMS group showed a significantly greater reduction in depression scores. A MANOVA for the CGI showed the same trend but failed to reach statistical significance (Wilks λ $F = 2.4$, $P = 0.09$).

The data were also analysed in a dichotomous fashion using a criterion of 50% reduction or more in MADRS or HDRS scores. In the TMS group 17 patients (49%) had a reduction of 50% or more on at least one of their depression rating scales, whereas only eight patients (25%) met this criterion in the sham-TMS group ($\chi^2 = 3.4$, df = 1, $P = 0.06$).

Questions

1. Was the study randomized and double-blind?   (15 marks)

2. Were there any important differences between the groups at baseline?   (15 marks)

3. What are the parameters F and df quoted in the text?

(10 marks)

4. What is a MANOVA? (10 marks)

5. What is the number needed to treat using a rating scale reduction of 50% on either the HDRS or the MADRS and on the CGI? Why were they all used? (30 marks)

6. What other study data might you wish to see before rTMS was used in your routine clinical practice? (20 marks)

Answers

1. Patients were randomized to treatment arms using computer-generated random numbers (5 marks). The patients were blinded to the use of sham treatment but it is not clear if the clinicians were blind (5 marks). The ratings were blind (5 marks), and this is sometimes part of a triple blind.

2. Yes. There were a higher number of melancholic features in patients allocated to the rTMS arm of the study (5 marks), who also had a more frequent diagnosis of major depressive disorder (5 marks). Both of these differences were statistically significant and could be important, as they suggest more severe illnesses, which may have reduced response in the rTMS-treated subjects (5 marks).

3. F is a test statistic used in an ANOVA (analysis of variance). It is the ratio of the between-groups variance to the within-groups variance (5 marks); df means degrees of freedom and is the number of independent comparisons in a data set (5 marks).

4. A multivariate analysis of variance is a parametric statistical test that compares two or more independent groups (5 marks) on the mean value of two or more dependent continuous variables simultaneously (5 marks).

5. Using the HDRS or MADRS, the CER = 25%, the EER = 49%. Therefore, the ARR = 24% (5 marks) and the NNT is 5 (rounded up to the nearest integer) (5 marks). Using the CGI the results are not given and are statistically insignificant (5 marks). They are all used because HDRS ratings are the standard measure of severity (5 marks), are more sensitive to

small changes (5 marks), the MADRS ratings and CGIs are used as clinically useful discrete measures (5 marks).

6. One would generally want to see data on adverse effects from this and other trials (5 marks), replication of effects in high-quality randomized double-blind placebo-controlled trials (5 marks), preferably including pragmatic trials/economic data/meta-analyses (5 marks each for up to two study types).

HARM/AETIOLOGY I

Read the following text taken from a paper (van Os & Selten 1998) in the *British Journal of Psychiatry* and answer the questions at the end of the paper.

Précis

The invasion and occupation of the Netherlands by the German army for 5 days in May 1940 was seen as a stressful national event. Individuals exposed to this stress in utero were compared with those who were born during the same time of the year in the 2-year periods before and after this event. The National Psychiatric Case Register, maintained since 1970, was used to follow up lifetime admissions to inpatient care within the Netherlands for schizophrenia in the two groups.

The results are given in Table 5.5.

Table 5.5   Incidence and relative risk of schizophrenia in those exposed to stress in utero compared with controls

	Cumulative incidence/1000 live births)		
	Exposed	Not exposed	Risk ratio (95%CI)
Combined	3.1	2.7	1.15 (1.03–1.28)
1st trimester	3.6	2.8	1.28 (1.07–1.53)
2nd trimester	2.9	2.6	1.09 (0.90–1.30)
3rd trimester	3.0	2.8	1.07 (0.88–1.30)

There was an interaction with gender in the second trimester-exposed cohorts (RR men: 1.35, 95%CI 1.05–1.74; RR women: 0.83, 95%CI 0.69–1.12).

Questions

1. What hypothesis did the researchers test? (10 marks)

2. What type of study is this? Explain your answer. (10 marks)

3. What is the other main method of studying the above issue? When would you use it? List two advantages and two disadvantages of this approach over a cohort study. (20 marks)

4. Where did the investigators obtain the data on the incidence of schizophrenia in each group? Describe two drawbacks to this approach. Can you suggest any modification to improve the accuracy of this technique? (15 marks)

5. Why and how did the investigators ensure the comparability of the follow-up duration between the groups? (10 marks)

6. Why did the investigators take special precautions to ensure that controls were in utero at the same time of year as the cases? (5 marks)

7. What is the risk ratio and how is it calculated? Are these risk ratios significant statistically? Are they clinically significant? Give reasons for your answers. (30 marks)

Answers

1. That exposure to stress in utero increases the risk of schizophrenia in later life (5 marks). Additional 5 marks if framed as a null hypothesis, i.e. that exposure to stress in utero does not increase the risk of schizophrenia in later life.

2. This is a controlled (2 marks), retrospective (2 marks) cohort study (2 marks), as the cases and controls were identified by their exposure status, but after the disease had occurred, and then followed forward in time. (4 marks for explanation)

3. The case–control study is the other main method of examining risk/harm (5 marks) A case–control study is the most economical method of studying rare outcomes or events (5 marks), whereas cohort studies are useful for studying rare exposures. The main advantages of a case–control study are that they are less time and resource consuming and can be used to study rare events (5 marks for any two advantages). The disadvantages include that they are generally more prone

to bias than are cohort studies (especially recall bias); the selection of an appropriate control group can be very difficult; one cannot infer causation (only association); and they can only be used to study a single outcome (5 marks for any two disadvantages).

4. The investigators went through the National Psychiatric Case Register from 1970 to the time of the study, to identify cases with a discharge diagnosis of schizophrenia (5 marks). Drawbacks include: may not identify cases with an onset pre 1970; would not identify late-onset cases; and would not identify cases that were never admitted (5 marks each for any two). The case finding could have been improved by attempting to corroborate the information from another source, e.g. subject interviews, contacting primary care physicians, etc. (5 marks for any one).

5. They ensured this comparability so that the cases and controls would have an equal chance of developing the disease of interest in the follow-up period, i.e. to reduce any bias introduced by uneven follow-up periods (5 marks). They did this by using control groups from a similar length of time both before and after the exposure, so that the total person-years of observation would be the same in cases and controls (5 marks).

6. The investigators wanted to make sure that no confounding could have been introduced by any seasonal variation in incidence. This has special significance for schizophrenia, as there is thought to be a higher incidence of winter births among those affected (5 marks).

7. The risk ratio, or relative risk, is the ratio of incidence among the exposed versus those not exposed (5 marks). Significance is determined by whether the 95%CI of the RR overlaps with one or not (5 marks for method only if subsequent answers are incorrect).

The following were statistically significant findings:

Combined cumulative incidence in exposed = 3.1; in non-exposed = 2.7; risk ratio = 1.15 (95%CI 1.03–1.28).

    First-trimester cumulative incidence in exposed = 3.6; in non-exposed = 2.8; risk ratio = 1.28 (95%CI 1.07–1.53).

(5 marks for both)

These findings were not statistically significant:

Second-trimester cumulative incidence in exposed = 2.9; in non-exposed = 2.6; risk ratio = 1.09 (95%CI = 0.90–1.30).

Third-trimester cumulative incidence in exposed = 3.0; in non-exposed = 2.8; risk ratio = 1.07 (95%CI = 0.88–1.30).

(5 marks for both)

The highest RR was only 1.28, i.e. those mothers exposed to pregnancy stress were 28% more likely to have offspring who later experienced schizophrenia (5 marks). However, clinical significance is more usefully measured using the number needed to harm (NNH). For children born to mothers who experienced maternal stress in the second trimester, the absolute risk increase is 3.6/1000–2.8/1000, or 0.8/1000. The NNH is the reciprocal of this figure and is equal to 1250 (5 marks). Therefore, because schizophrenia is fairly rare, 1250 mothers needed to be exposed to maternal stress to bring about one extra case of schizophrenia in their offspring. Arguably this is clinically insignificant (5 marks).

HARM/AETIOLOGY II

Read the following excerpt from a published paper (Sadowski et al 1999) and answer the questions at the end.

Précis

This study randomly selected 296 from an original sample of 1000 who were participants in the Newcastle Thousand Family Study in the first 5 years of their life. The original sample underwent assessment up to the first 15 years of life, and the following six family disadvantages were defined in the first 5 years of life: family/marital disruption; parental physical illness; poor physical care of the child and home; social dependence (serious debts, unemployment, etc.); family overcrowding; and poor mothering. The 296 individuals were selected from three strata: those not disadvantaged; those with one or two disadvantages; and those with three or more disadvantages. In this phase of the study it was decided to focus on a more stringent definition of multiple disadvantage based on the mean and standard deviation of disadvantages in the sample. The participants were dichotomized as follows: (a) 'no multiple disadvantages' ($n = 257$, 85.3%), and 'those experiencing up to three coexisting disadvantages; and (b) 'multiple disadvantage' ($n = 39$, 14.7%), i.e. those experiencing at least four coexisting family criteria of disadvantages in their first 5 years of life. The subjects were interviewed in their 33rd year of life. Outcome assessment was done by interviewers trained in structured assessments using a standard protocol. They were blind to the subjects' pasts or disadvantages. The assessment involved a retrospective view of the past 1 year for affective and anxiety symptoms. Multiple logistic regression analysis was used to study the influence of disadvantages on the outcome using backwards-stepwise selection.

The results are summarized in Table 5.6.

Table 5.6 Risk factors for later symptoms of anxiety and depression

Risk factors	Adjusted odds ratio (95%CI)
Multiple disadvantages at the age of 5 years	2.2 (1.4–3.4) SE = 1
Female gender	1.6 (1.0–2.5) SE = 0.75
Family or marital instability	1.7 (1.1–2.8) SE = 0.85
Social dependence and overcrowding	2.0 (1.2–3.3) SE = 1.05
Poor physical care of the child and poor mothering	3.1 (1.0–9.1) SE = 4.05
Poor physical care, poor mothering and female sex	1.8 (1.1–2.9) SE = 0.9

Questions

1. What advantages does a cohort study have over case–control studies in assessing aetiology/harm? Does it have any drawbacks? (10 marks)

2. Comment on the sample selection. Was it randomized and representative? What is the term used for this sampling technique? (15 marks)

3. Six areas of psychosocial disadvantages were selected. Can you mention two confounding factors that could affect this study and appear as a family disadvantage? How can they confound the results? (15 marks)

4. Inspect the category list of family disadvantages in the first 5 years of life and suggest two ways in which two or more of these may be linked. What is the statistical term for such variables? (15 marks)

5. How did the raters assess the outcome? Mention two ways in which their method tried to reduce biases in assessments. Explain how each of these could improve the rating. Describe one way in which the diagnosis may be missed and how this could have been prevented. (20 marks)

6. Arrange the odds ratios in order of their precision. Explain how you did this. (15 marks)

7. The authors used multiple logistic regression analysis in this study. State briefly what this technique aims to do. What statistical technique can be used to reduce complex, large data sets to a smaller number of explanatory variables? (10 marks)

Answers

1. Advantages: (a) A cohort study is a prospective design and therefore not subject to recall biases as are case–control studies. (b) The outcome is not known in cohort studies and observation bias (in favour of the better-outcome group) can be reduced. (c) The technique is most economical when rare exposures are being measured. Drawbacks: (a) If the event of interest is rare cohort studies may not identify them all. (b) Cohort studies are more time, labour and cost intensive (5 marks for two advantages, 5 marks for two disadvantages).

2. The sample was selected for a cohort from the Newcastle Thousand Family Study (5 marks). The method of selection was randomized and therefore likely to be representative of the group as a whole (5 marks). Sampling was done by selecting from three different groups within the original cohort. This is an example of stratified random sampling (5 marks).

3. Examples of confounding factors:
   (a) Chronic physical illness or disability in the child.
   (b) Mental or behavioural problems in the child.
   (c) Childhood traumas, physical or mental, that arose from outside the family environment (5 marks each = 10 marks for any two, or any other possible confounders).

   The above constitute factors which may be outside the control of the family, may make the child more vulnerable, and even lead to adversity as defined in the paper (e.g. family disruption/marital disharmony). If missed these would falsely strengthen the association between family adversity and adult depression (5 marks).

4. (a) Poor mothering can be a result of parental illness.
   (b) Family disruption, family overcrowding and social dependence can all lead to poor care of the child.
   (c) Marital disruption can be a result of overcrowding, social dependence and parental illness (5 marks for one, 10 marks for any two).
   Linked factors like these are called confounders (5 marks).

5. The raters conducted face-to-face interviews to assess depression.

   The following methods were used to decrease bias: the raters were trained (this would improve interrater reliability); a structured protocol was used (this would also improve interrater reliability); raters were blind to the subjects' past family adversity (this would decrease any biases in rating those with more adversity as more unwell) (5 marks for each, to a maximum of 10 marks).

   The rating scale used assessed depressive symptoms in the past 1 year; episodes before that may be missed. A lifetime diagnosis would have been more appropriate (5 marks). Some of the 'well' subjects may subsequently develop depression. This can be picked up by prospective follow-ups over reasonable intervals of time, e.g. 5 years (5 marks).

6. The order of precision of the odds ratios is:
   1 Female sex
   2 Family or marital instability
   3 Poor physical care of the child, poor mothering and female sex
   4 Multiple disadvantages at the age of 5 years
   5 Social dependence and overcrowding
   6 Poor physical care of the child and poor mothering
   (10 marks for all correct, 5 marks if one mistake)

   Increasing precision is associated with narrower confidence intervals and smaller standard errors (5 marks).

7. Logistic regression analysis is used to study the influence of several independent variables on dichotomous outcomes (5 marks). A principal component analysis could have been used to reduce the variables into common factors (5 marks).

PROGNOSIS I

The following text is taken from a published paper by Duggan et al (1998). Read it carefully and answer the questions at the end.

Précis

The family history of 89 consecutive patients with an RDC diagnosis of major depression was collected: 116, 283 and 120 first-degree relatives were examined using SADS-L, FH-RDC and case notes, respectively. The outcome of 74 (83%) of the patients was examined. The presence of a severe psychiatric illness (suicide, hospitalized depression and psychosis) was associated with a poor outcome. This association persisted after correction for family size, age structure and gender using logistic regression analysis. The family history did not correlate with Kendell's neurotic psychotic index or the proband's neuroticism scores.

Table 5.7 Outcomes of major depression disorder by number of affected relatives

N. of affected relatives	Good outcome group (n = 25)	Poor outcome group (n = 49)
0	21	29
1	4	14
2	0	4
3	0	1
4	0	1

Questions

1. The authors in this study are looking for prognostic features in depressive illness. How is a prognostic factor different from a risk factor? (10 marks)

2. List the different types of study that can be used reliably to study prognosis. (15 marks)

3. What method was used to define outcome in this study? What are your comments about its adequacy? Give three characteristics of good outcome measurement in a prognosis study. (25 marks)

4. The authors have used different methods to collect the family history. What are your comments about this? What additional precaution should they take to prevent bias in assessments?

(15 marks)

5. Use the figures given in Table 5.7 to construct a contingency (2 × 2) table to calculate odds ratios. What are the odds of a poor outcome with a family history of a severe mental illness? Now calculate the odds ratio for a poor outcome for patients with, rather than without, a family history of illness. How do you interpret this?   (20 marks)

6. What did the authors achieve by controlling for family size, age and gender? Explain the significance with reference to each of these terms (15 marks).

Answers

1. Prognostic factors predict outcomes (5 marks), whereas strictly speaking risk factors are linked directly with disease causation, for example smoking and lung cancer (5 marks).

2. (a) Cohort study.
   (b) Case–control studies.
   (c) Randomized controlled trial.   (5 marks each: 15 marks)

3. 'Severe psychiatric illness' was used to define the outcome categories (5 marks). These criteria are not defined in this paper and their reliability and validity are not known (5 marks). Ideally outcome measure should:
   (a) be objective (5 marks)
   (b) have good interrater reliability of the measure (5 marks)
   (c) be applied blindly, i.e. without the knowledge of the presence or absence of particular prognostic factors (5 marks).

4. First-degree relatives ($n = 116$, 283 and 120) were examined using SADS-L, FH-RDC and case notes, respectively. This is a reasonably comprehensive method (5 marks), but data particularly from case notes can be subject to recording bias (poor recall, omitted entries, etc.) (5 marks). The persons involved in the collection of family history should be blind to the patients' outcome or they may be biased in detecting more severe illnesses in families of those with poor outcomes (5 marks).

5. Contingency table

	Poor outcome	Good outcome	
Family history	20	4	
No family history	29	21	
	49	25	Total = 74

(5 marks if all entries correct)

Odds of a poor outcome with family history of illness = 20/4 = 5:1 (5 marks)

Odds of a poor outcome without family history of illness = 29/21 = 1.38

Odds ratio of a poor outcome with, compared to without, family history of illness = ratio of the odds calculated above = 5/1.38 = 3.62 (5 marks)

Interpretation: Patients with a family history of mental illness are three to four times more likely to have a poor outcome than not, compared with patients without a family history (5 marks).

6. The authors made sure that the initial differences between the groups with respect to these factors did not confound the results (5 marks for method if other parts of question are incorrect).

Family size: A patient with larger family has more chance of a family member being affected than does one with a smaller family (5 marks).

Age: A patient with older relatives is more likely to have affected relatives simply because the illness has had time to manifest (5 marks).

Gender: The gender of the patient may have an influence on outcome, e.g. more male suicide (5 marks).

PROGNOSIS II

Read the following article based on a published paper of O'Brien et al (1998) and answer the questions at the end.

Précis

Sixty depressed subjects over the age of 55 were selected from consecutive admissions of two psychiatric and two general hospital units. DSM-III R was used to diagnose major depression. The Hamilton Depression Rating Scale and the Cambridge cognitive examination (CAMDEX) were used for baseline assessment. The subjects underwent baseline T_2-weighted MRI scans which were rated blindly by two raters using a standard 0–3 scale. Deep white matter lesions (WML) and periventricular white matter lesions were examined. The κ values for the ratings were 0.75 for periventricular WML and 0.8 for deep WML. When raters disagreed the rating made by one of the raters was used consistently. Experienced blind raters performed follow-up. All baseline assessments were repeated (except MRI), and data were also collected from notes, clinical follow-up and informants. Mean follow-up was 31.9 (9.9) months. Six subjects refused follow-up, one died after 2 months; eight subjects were followed up for 12–24 months, 20 for 24–36 months and 25 for 36 months or more. A Kaplan–Meier survival analysis was performed on the data. As far as possible annual follow-ups were planned based on clinical need. Periventricular white matter lesions were not associated with outcome. Deep WML were associated with outcome after age, sex, duration of depression before initial assessment, age at onset and cardiovascular risk factors were taken into account. Fisher's exact probability test was used for comparison between good and bad outcomes. Table 5.8 summarizes the results.

Table 5.8 Outcome of depression in those with (severe/moderate) and without (mild/none) deep white matter lesions (DWML)

	DWML+		DWML–	
	n (%)	95%CI	*n* (%)	95%CI
Continuously well	0 (0)	0–21	11 (27)	14–43
Recovered	1 (8)	0–36	7 (17)	7–32
Continuously ill	6 (46)	19–75	14 (34)	20–51
Demented/died	6 (46)	19–75	9 (22)	11–38
Total	13		41	

Questions

1. Summarize the objective of the study. How would you design the study if you wanted to study white matter lesions as a risk factor rather than a prognostic factor in depression? (15 marks)

2. How were the MRI white matter lesions rated? Enumerate two strong points of the study with respect to this. Mention one apparent weakness in the assessment. (15 marks)

3. How were the follow-ups planned and what drawback do you see in this? What sources of information were used? What did the investigators do to prevent bias in the follow-up design? (15 marks)

4. What was the dropout rate in the first year? Why have the authors used survival analysis techniques? What is survival analysis? (20 marks)

5. Extract data from the table of results and display as a 2×2 table for a good or poor outcome. Calculate the odds of poor outcome with severe and not-severe lesions. Calculate the odds ratio of poor outcome with deep white matter lesions. (20 marks)

6. The authors have used Fisher's exact probability test. What is the purpose of this? When is this test particularly indicated? (10 marks)

7. How did the authors handle confounding factors in the outcome? (5 marks)

Answers

1. Are white matter lesions (WML) in MRI a prognostic factor in the elderly with major depressive disorder? (5 marks)

   For study of WML as risk factor, normal elderly subjects would need to undergo MRI scanning to select a cohort who have severe WML and those who do not (5 marks). The cohorts would then need to be followed up for a sufficient length of time to calculate the risk of depression in each group (5 marks).

2. MRI lesions were rated as deep and periventricular and within each category as severe or moderate, mild or no lesions (5 marks). Strengths: two independent raters were used, raters

were blind to the diagnosis, and a standard rating scale was used to rate the lesions (5 marks for any two). Weaknesses: Ratings of one person were given preference if there were disagreements: an explicit method for deciding which rater's measurements took preference is not stated (5 marks for any one).

3. Follow-ups were planned annually. The drawback is that they were according to clinical circumstances, and therefore some patients would have been followed up more often than others. This may result in their being assigned poorer ratings irrespective of the actual clinical severity of illness (5 marks).

   Follow-up data derived from: clinical interviews, rating using Hamilton Depression Rating Scale and CAMDEX, information from case notes and information from informants (5 marks). Raters were blind to findings of the MRI to prevent bias in follow-up ratings (5 marks).

4. The dropout rate was 10% (6/60) (5 marks). Survival analysis was used as the patients had different periods of follow-up (5 marks). When subjects are followed for different periods of time, or not followed long enough to observe the events of interest, a survival analysis is done. This calculates the probable number of subjects who would survive (or not have the event of interest, such as depression in this example) over the period of time considered (5 marks). This can be depicted as a survival curve, also called a Kaplan–Meier curve (5 marks).

5. Contingency table

Lesion	Poor outcome	Good outcome	
DWML+	12	1	
DWML−	23	18	
	35	19	Total = 54

(5 marks if all entries correct)

Odds of poor outcome with DWML+ = 12/1 = 12 (5 marks)
Odds of poor outcome with DWML− = 23/18 = 1.27 (5 marks)
Odds ratio = 12/1.27 = 9.45 (5 marks)

6. Fisher's exact probability test is used to compare two proportions (or to compare observed with expected

frequencies) for categorical data organized into a 2 × 2 table
(5 marks) when the cell sizes are small (5 marks). It calculates
the probability that the numbers in each cell of the table could
have occurred by chance alone.

7. The authors performed an analysis to predict the influence of
confounding variables such as age, sex, duration of depression,
and cardiovascular risk factors. These were not significantly
associated with outcome (5 marks).

SYSTEMATIC REVIEW I

Read the following précis of a published article and answer the
questions at the end.

Précis

The Cochrane Dementia and Cognitive Impairment Group
Register of Clinical Trials was searched using the terms
'donepezil', 'E2020' and 'ARICEPT'. MEDLINE, PsychLit and
EMBASE electronic databases were also searched with the above
terms. Members of the Donepezil Study Group and Eisai Inc.
were contacted. All unconfounded, double-blind randomized
controlled trials in which treatment with donepezil was
administered for more than a day and compared with placebo in
patients with Alzheimer's disease were selected. Data were
extracted independently by the reviewers, pooled where
appropriate and possible, and the weighted or standardized mean
differences or Peto odds ratios (95%CI) estimated. Where
possible, intention-to-treat data were used. Four trials met the
criteria, covering treatment of 12 or 24 weeks' duration in highly
selected patients. The only information available on one trial
(Gauthier 1998) is a conference abstract which reports no useable
results. Available outcome data cover domains including cognitive
function and global clinical state, but data on several important
dimensions of outcome are not available. There were significantly
more withdrawals before the end of treatment from the 10 mg/day
(but not the 5 mg/day) donepezil group compared with placebo,
which may have resulted in some overestimation of beneficial
changes at 10 mg/day in progressively declining characteristics, as
last available measures were used in the analyses. A variety of

adverse effects were recorded, but very few patients left a trial as a direct result of the intervention.

Table 5.9   Therapeutic effects of 5 and 10 mg doses of donepezil compared with placebo

Results	5 mg (95%CI)	10 mg (95%CI)
(WMD) in ADAS-COG scores	−2.6 (−3.5, −1.8)	−3.0 (−3.9, −2.1)
Peto OR for global clinical state improvement	0.4 (0.3, 0.62)	0.4 (0.3, 0.6)
Quality of life WMD	7.1 (−4.5, 18.7)	0.04 (17.0, 17.0)

In selected patients with mild or moderate Alzheimer's disease treated for periods of 12 or 24 weeks, donepezil produced modest improvements in cognitive function, and study clinicians rated global clinical state more positively in treated patients. No significant effect on patient self-assessed quality of life was found.

Questions

1. Define the term meta-analysis and systematic review.

(10 marks)

2. How did the authors ensure that they did not miss any relevant trials? Comment with reference to their search strategy. Is there any way the strategy could be made more robust? (15 marks)

3. In a systematic review what can lead to lack of reporting of trials? How can this be assessed? Describe two methods.

(15 marks)

4. What did the authors do to assess the quality of the papers in the trial? Can you suggest any modifications to make the check more rigorous? (10 marks)

5. What is meant by dichotomous outcome measure and what is its importance in interpreting the data? Why is it used clinically? (15 marks)

6. Look at the results given above. Define the term weighted mean difference? Why do you think the WMD for quality of life ratings at the 10 mg dose is not significant, although the

actual difference is large? Comment on the precision of the estimate. (20 marks)

7. Can this study be generalized to all patients with Alzheimer's disease? Mention two reasons for choosing and two for not choosing this treatment in practice. (15 marks)

Answers

1. Systematic reviews are comprehensive reviews of research work, selected using prespecified explicit criteria (5 marks). Meta-analysis is the statistical summary of the studies weighted for quality and/or precision (5 marks).

2. The authors searched several electronic databases using specific search terms. They also wrote to researchers and the drug company (5 marks). The strategy can be improved by searching more databases and by performing a hand search of important and relevant journals for trials of donepezil in Alzheimer's disease (5 marks). References from the articles selected can be another source of information (5 marks).

3. Publication biases can lead to lack of reporting. Small positive studies are more likely to be published than data from small negative trials. Therefore, publication bias tends to overestimate the beneficial effects of treatment (5 marks).

   Funnel plot analysis looks specifically for publication bias in reporting or publishing the trial. A funnel plot involves plotting the study size against the odds ratios. Any biases in reporting will skew the normally symmetrical shape of the plot (5 marks). A Galbraith plot can be used to generate a P value for publication bias, although it needs some adaptation to perform this function (5 marks).

4. Preset criteria were used to assess the quality of trials according to blinding, confounding and randomization (5 marks). Blinding both investigators to the source and authorship of the papers and measuring their interrater reliability can improve the quality assessment (5 marks).

5. A dichotomous outcome measure splits the results into two categories, e.g. improved/not improved, or affected/not affected (5 marks). This division helps increase the ease of clinical interpretation and application, allowing statistics such

as absolute risk reduction, relative risk reduction, odds ratios and NNTs to be calculated (5 marks). Dichotomous outcome measures are often preferred to continuous ones clinically, as clinical decisions also tend to be dichotomous (treat/don't treat, admit/don't admit, etc.) (5 marks).

6. Weighted mean difference: The difference between scores of the placebo and the donepezil group is adjusted by attaching weights based on standard error of the scores (5 marks). These values are then pooled to give a weighted mean difference (5 marks).

   Even though 7.1 is a large difference, the confidence interval for this difference crosses 0 and is therefore not statistically significant (5 marks). The confidence interval is very large, indicating that the standard error is large and the precision low (5 marks).

7. No, this study can be applied only to mild and moderately affected patients and not to the severely ill (5 marks).

   Possible reasons for choosing donepezil:

   (a) It improves cognitive function.
   (b) It improves the functioning of patients.

   (5 marks)

   Possible reasons for not choosing donepezil:

   (c) Patients do not perceive any change in quality of life.
   (d) The improvement in cognitive function is small, even if significant. (5 marks)

SYSTEMATIC REVIEW II

Read the following text adapted from a published paper (Hulse et al 1998) and answer the questions at the end.

Précis

English-language articles were identified using MEDLINE. Articles were also selected from the references in those articles. Only studies that had control groups were selected. Seven studies were included in the analysis, which looked specifically for risk in women who were switched to methadone early in pregnancy, women who were switched to methadone later in pregnancy, and women who continued to use heroin along with methadone during pregnancy. None of the studies was controlled for confounding variables, though some showed poor antenatal care with heroin use (no figures supplied). The common odds test was used as a test of homogeneity. In the calculation of pooled effect sizes a random effects model was applied where homogeneity figures were low and a fixed effect model was used where heterogeneity was low. The relative risk estimate for neonatal mortality for separate heroin and methadone use was close to unity. The overall results for heroin use were probably unduly influenced by a single large study which, unlike the smaller studies, found a relative risk near unity. Analysis was also repeated after the removal of this study. The pooled estimate of relative risk (RR) is given below. It may well be that the chaotic lifestyle associated with heroin and methadone use contributed to a high risk ratio.

Table 5.10 Relative risk of neonatal mortality by maternal opiate use

Opiate type	RR (95% CI)
Heroin	3.27 (0.95–9.60)
Methadone	1.75 (0.60–2.33)
Heroin and methadone	6.37 (2.57–14.68)
Any methadone	3.00 (1.50–5.88)
Any opiate	2.55 (1.89–3.38)

Questions

1. Frame your question for a search, clearly describing the clinical issues involved in this scenario.   (5 marks)

2. The authors of this paper searched MEDLINE. Name three important electronic databases they could have searched for studies. What is the advantage of searching more databases? Describe two other ways to obtain relevant studies. (15 marks)

3. Why did the authors not include other kinds of study, i.e. case reports, non-randomized and non-controlled trials? Give two reasons. When should one use such studies?   (15 marks)

4. The authors report that none of the studies controlled for confounding variables. Can you name three possible confounding variables in this study?   (10 marks)

5. Tests of homogeneity were applied to the papers. What are tests of homogeneity? What methods of statistical summary should be used when heterogeneity is high or low?   (10 marks)

6. What is relative risk? Why is the relative risk of opiate use and methadone use not considered significant in Table 5.10?
(10 marks)

7. The authors removed a study and recalculated the figures for relative risk due to heroin use. What was different about the removed study and what is the name given to this type of analysis?
(10 marks)

8. The authors report chaotic lifestyle as possibly being responsible for the high risk ratios. Is this statement justified? What should have been done to study the influence of lifestyle on neonatal mortality?   (10 marks)

9. Recently meta-analysis of observational studies has attracted a lot of criticism. Give two reasons why this might be the case, compared with a meta-analysis of randomized controlled trials.
(15 marks)

Answers

1. Is *opiate use* in *pregnancy* associated with increased *neonatal mortality compared with placebo/other opiate* (5 marks)? The terms in italics are part of a four-part clinical question that can be used to search for relevant information.

2. EMBASE, PsychLit, Cochrane Collaboration database (5 marks for any two). Electronic databases have biases in listing papers, and the use of more than one database may increase the identification of relevant papers (5 marks). Writing to the experts in the field and to companies manufacturing opiate drugs may also help identify further published and unpublished studies (5 marks).

3. Case reports and non-randomized or non-controlled trials come lower in the hierarchy of evidence (5 marks). Methodological differences will prevent a systematic review with such data (5 marks). These can be used to offer evidence in the absence of randomized controlled trials (5 marks).

4. (a) Abuse of other drugs such as alcohol and nicotine.
   (b) Coexisting poor nutrition.
   (c) Poor attention to medical problems. (10 marks for any two)

5. Tests of homogeneity are applied to studies in a systematic review. They indicate whether the variation in the results of studies is greater than would be expected by chance alone (5 marks). Testing for homogeneity helps in the interpretation of results, for example low homogeneity/high heterogeneity could lead to biased results in favour of the papers with large sample sizes. Statistical analysis/models can be chosen depending on the level of heterogeneity. Fixed effects analysis is the name given to the statistical summary of several studies where heterogeneity is low, and random effects analysis is generally used where there is evidence of heterogeneity (5 marks). In practice, however, tests for heterogeneity are low in power and both models are usually employed.

6. Relative risk is the ratio of the risk of an outcome in those exposed to an agent to the risk of the outcome in those unexposed (5 marks). Table 5.10 shows RR for methadone and heroin use as 3.27 and 1.75 respectively; however, the confidence interval crosses unity, indicating that the result is not statistically significant (5 marks).

7. In this case the larger study showed a relative risk close to unity (5 marks). The authors removed this study presumably because they thought it was clinically or statistically heterogeneous. This manipulation is a type of sensitivity analysis (5 marks).

8. The authors have not shown any lifestyle-related risk figures. Therefore, they are not justified in making this assumption (5 marks). Lifestyle may influence neonatal mortality and some of the studies did study the effect of regular follow-up and mortality. However, chaotic lifestyle should have been defined operationally before the analysis was done and included as criteria for study selection (5 marks).

9. Meta-analyses of observational studies are criticized because they give weaker evidence than that from randomized controlled trials and other studies that are further up the evidence hierarchy (see section on clinical practice guideline

for details) (5 marks). They are therefore more likely to be subject to bias and confounding and may produce spuriously precise results, though this is somewhat debatable (10 marks for any two points).

ECONOMICS I

Read the following abridged paper (Kraft et al 1998) carefully and then answer questions 1–8 at the end. You may find it easier to read the questions first.

Précis

A group of 100 methadone-maintained opiate users were randomly assigned to three treatment groups receiving different levels of support services during a 24-week clinical trial. One group received minimal counselling at a rate of once per month ($n = 31$). A second group received counselling at a rate of three times per week plus behavioural interventions ($n = 36$). The third group received enhanced support in the form of seven counselling sessions per week, plus extended on-site medical, psychiatric, employment and family therapy services ($n = 33$). During the 6-month follow-up period all patients continued to receive the counselling-and-methadone level of treatment.

All subjects received between 60 and 90 mg/day of methadone. No ancillary medications, counselling or other professional services were provided, except in emergency circumstances. All subjects were administered the Addiction Severity Index upon admission to the programme, at the end of the 24-week clinical trial, and at the 6-month follow-up. Four types of variable were required to construct the 12-month cost-effectiveness ratio:

1. Salary and benefits of the professional staff.
2. Average direct and indirect contact time per treatment episode.
3. Number and type of service contacts per client.
4. Client outcome measures.

The salaries and benefits of the professional staff were derived from the Veterans Administration (VA) personnel reports based on 1993 figures. The average time spent performing various types of service activity was determined by a panel of drug treatment specialists, and by interviews with staff members at the Philadelphia VA methadone programme.

Outcome measures, collected at the 6-month follow-up with use of the Addiction Severity Index, were the same as those assessed at baseline and at the end of 12 weeks. They included medical needs, welfare dependency, days of illegal activity, illegal income, psychological problems, drug use and increased unemployment.

The cost per client to achieve a certain outcome measure was constructed by using the cost of services per client for the 24-week trial period, plus the cost of service for 6 months of methadone plus counselling as the index numerator. The denominator was the drug abstinence rate at follow-up. An additional economic analysis was performed to provide policy makers with information on programme size or the optimum number of treatment slots. The marginal cost analysis gives the cost required to achieve an outcome of abstinence in one additional client.

Table 5.11   Characteristics of methadone study subjects at baseline

Variable	Minimum services	Intermediate services	Enhanced services	F or χ^2	P
Age (yrs)	42.3	41.8	43.4	0.71	0.49
Heroin use	12.3	12.3	11.9	0.41	0.67
Male (%)	83.9	83.3	87.9	0.26	0.88
Married (%)	25.8	25	18.2	0.65	0.72

At 24 weeks, subjects in the enhanced methadone services group showed significantly better outcomes, as measured by urine screening and the Addiction Severity Index, than the clients receiving counselling plus methadone services and minimum methadone services, with respect to decreases in medical needs, welfare dependency, days of illegal activity, illegal income, psychological problems, drug use and increased unemployment. However, at 12 months – 6 months after supplemental services were stopped – only the difference in the level of abstinence from heroin remained statistically significant across groups ($F = 4.05$, df = 2.97, $P = 0.02$), although there was no statistically significant difference between the intermediate and intensive groups in terms of the level of abstinence.

At 52 weeks, when the long-term assessment was performed, abstinence rates had declined in all groups, from 30% to 29% in the minimal intervention group, from 55% to 47% in the counselling plus methadone services group, and from 68% to 49% in the enhanced methadone services group.

At 12 months, with the use of mean cost values, the annual cost per abstinent client was estimated as $16,485 for minimum methadone services, $9,804 for counselling plus methadone services, and $11,818 for enhanced methadone services.

Questions

1. What sort of study is this? (10 marks)

2. Name two limitations of this study. (10 marks)

3. What does a cost-effectiveness analysis aim to do? (10 marks)

4. What other types of economic study do you know and what are their aims? (20 marks)

5. How many people do you need to treat with intensive counselling to bring about one patient with a superior outcome compared with intermediate counselling at 12 months? (10 marks)

6. How might the authors have checked their results to see whether they were robust to minor changes in the costs and outcomes used? What types of this analysis are you aware of? (20 marks)

7. How would you explain to the managers of your hospital the findings of this study? (10 marks)

8. Why does Table 5.11 give 'F or χ^2' values? (10 marks)

Answers

1. This is a cost-effectiveness study that examines the cost per unit health improvement (5 marks). The study is based on a clinical trial of methadone maintenance plus three different levels of additional care. The study is randomized and controlled, but patients and clinicians are not blind to which treatment is being received (5 marks).

2. Three main disadvantages (not exhaustive): The study may yield data inferior to a double-blind randomized controlled

trial (less internal validity), giving a less accurate estimate of treatment efficacy. The main outcome considered is abstinence, but there may have been many other important outcomes which were not considered, such as crime. Furthermore, the use of quality-adjusted life years may have been a more suitable design, as they can compare treatments when the benefits are measured in many different and otherwise incompatible units (5 marks for any two from the above or any other reasonable criticism).

3. A cost-effectiveness analysis aims to show which treatment provides the greatest healthcare benefit per unit cost (5 marks). The cost per healthcare benefit can be compared directly or, when a treatment is both more effective and more expensive, the incremental cost may be useful (5 marks), (i.e. where the amount of additional cost per extra unit of healthcare improvement is calculated).

4. The other main types of economic evaluation are:
   Cost–benefit: This is where treatment costs and consequences are compared in the same monetary units. It can be useful especially where the health improvement cannot be converted into equal units by any other method (10 marks).

   Cost–utility: This is where the consequences of treatments are considered in utility units. The most common way of performing this type of study is in terms of the cost per QALY (quality-adjusted life year) gained (10 marks).

5. A treatment question.
   At 12 months CER = 47%, EER = 49%; therefore, ARR = 2% and NNT = 50 (5 marks each for ARR and NNT).

6. The authors could have performed a sensitivity analysis to see if their conclusions were robust to changes in the costs and consequences of treatment (5 marks). The most common way of doing this is by a one-way sensitivity analysis, where the costs and consequences are varied one at a time to calculate the critical values at which the study conclusions would change (5 marks). The next most robust method of sensitivity analysis is an 'extreme scenario analysis' (5 marks). Perhaps the most robust method is the Monte Carlo sensitivity analysis. This is where several parameters are varied together, and is quoted as one of the most rigorous methods of sensitivity analysis (5 marks).

7. I would explain to the managers that although intensive counselling produces more abstinent users short term, this is not sustained (5 marks). Intermediate services are comparable to lower levels of care at 12 months in terms of efficacy, and are less expensive per successfully treated patient than either more or less intensive alternatives (5 marks). (Incremental costs per abstinent could be calculated, although differences in abstinence rates were not statistically significant and the much larger costs of the enhanced regimen would mean that incremental costs are likely to be high.)

8. F or χ^2 are tests of statistical significance. F is used where data are continuous, and is the test statistic when an analysis of variance is used (5 marks). χ^2 is given where data are categorical and is used to compare observed with expected frequencies (5 marks).

ECONOMICS II

Read the following abridged paper (Creed et al 1997) carefully and then answer questions 1–9 at the end.

The paper studies the cost-effectiveness of day versus inpatient psychiatric treatment. It is adapted from a paper published in the *British Medical Journal*.

Précis

For over a decade the Manchester Royal Infirmary's psychiatric day hospital has treated acutely ill patients as an alternative to inpatient treatment . Day patient and inpatient treatment has led to similar social and clinical outcomes.

This paper compares the costs of day and inpatient treatment. Day hospital treatment for acutely ill patients may place an excessive burden on the carers, and so costs to family members were included both as monetary and non-monetary variables.

This study was conducted over 3 years. Randomization was conducted by randomly sorting cards in sealed envelopes, to be opened by an independent administrator. After randomization clinicians managed the patients as usual, determining discharge dates and readmissions independent of the researchers.

All patients aged ´18–65 years presenting to the service for admission were considered for the study. Exclusions were compulsory admissions or patients too ill for day treatment; patients discharged in under 5 days; admissions solely for detoxification of drugs and alcohol; and patients with a diagnosis of organic brain disease, personality disorder or mania. Psychiatric diagnosis was assessed at admission with the present state examination (PM and BW), and the severity of the psychiatric symptoms was measured with the comprehensive psychopathological rating scale at admission and after 3 and 12 months. Disturbed behaviour after admission was assessed with the modified social behaviour schedule, completed by the patient's key nurse. Distress in carers was also assessed using the general health questionnaire (GHQ).

Direct costs to the Trust: The duration of the first and any subsequent inpatient or day patient admissions, number and length of interviews with medical staff and community psychiatric nurses, and investigations at the hospital were costed at local rates. Costs to the mental health service in Manchester, including 'hotel' and staffing costs, were identified down to unit of service. The costs of drugs were based on *British National Formulary* figures, adjusted to take account of overheads. Day hospital admissions were costed (staffing and overheads) by using the number of days that patients actually attended the hospital.

Direct costs to other agencies: These were costed on information from the records of general practitioners and social workers. Costs of visits were based on national unit costs of community care, as detailed local information was not available.

Indirect costs to other agencies: These were estimated from interviews with the main carer. The carer recalled travelling costs related to the patient's illness, and an estimate was also made of increased household expenditure and reduction in the patient's or carer's income. The time that the patient and carer spent travelling and in outpatient and other departments during appointments was estimated, but could not be costed. The average time per day that the carer spent in direct care of the patient (while ill) was also estimated and expressed in hours per day.

All the above monetary costs were adjusted to 1994–1995 prices by using the relevant price index. During the second half of the study additional support was provided to help the treatment of acutely ill day patients. A community psychiatric nurse was available on call during evenings and weekends. This increased patient contacts with the CPNs but did not significantly affect overall costs.

Data analysis and statistics

An intention-to-treat analysis compared inpatient and outpatient treatment groups. Clinical and social outcome costs were compared over 12 months after the first admission.

Ninety-three inpatients and 94 day patients were randomized. Eight were excluded because of early discharge or diagnosis, leaving 89 inpatients and 90 day patients. Five randomly selected inpatients were transferred to the day hospital because of lack of beds, and 11 day patients were transferred to the inpatient unit because they were too ill for the day hospital; 104 patients (52 inpatients, 52 day patients) had a resident carer who was available for repeated interviews.

At admission inpatients and day patients showed no significant differences in sex, mean age, ethnic origin, employment status, marital status, and diagnosis or illness severity.

Clinical and social outcome

Scores for psychiatric symptoms, social behaviour and role performance were all significantly reduced 6 and 12 months after admission, and there was no significant difference between day patients and inpatients at these times. At 2 and 4 weeks inpatients showed fewer psychiatric symptoms and abnormal behaviours, indicating more rapid recovery than day patients. Social behaviour assessment schedule scores were lower at 12 months in the day patient group, indicating that they were less of a burden to carers at that time. GHQ scores were not significantly different at any time.

Resource use and costs

Direct costs: Randomized inpatients accumulated a mean of 62 inpatient days and seven day-hospital days over the 12 months. For day patients the figures were 32 day-hospital days and 21 inpatient days. The duration of interview with medical staff (11 versus 10 hours) was similar, but day patients spent more time with CPNs ($P<0.05$). Costs of hospital investigation and drugs were similar. The median overall difference in costs to CMHT was £1923 less for day patients. Direct costs to other agencies showed no significant differences. Loss of patients' income through illness, absences from work or unemployment was similar. Not surprisingly, patients' travelling costs were highest for the day hospital group ($P<0.05$). Total costs given monetary value showed day hospital treatment to be significantly cheaper (median difference £2165, 95%CI £737–£3593).

Table 5.12   Comprehensive Psychopathological Rating Scale symptom scores and social behaviour scores at admission and at 1-year follow-up

	Inpatients		Day patients		Difference	P value
	Mean	**Number**	**Mean**	**Number**		
Comprehensive rating scale score						
Admission	23.0	87	25.4	89	−2.3	0.13
1 year	8.6	65	7.2	67	1.4	0.44
Social behaviour						
Admission	16.62	52	18.06	51	−1.44	0.43
1 year	7.78	44	6.72	46	1.06	0.44

Cost to carers: There was a significantly greater loss of income among the carers of day hospital patients, primarily as a result of two carers becoming unemployed. Travel costs were significantly greater for the carers of inpatients. When all direct and indirect costs to patients and carers were considered, the median costs for day hospital were £1994 less than for inpatient treatment (95%CI £600–£3543).

Time spent travelling was significantly greater for day patients, but carers' travelling time and outpatient and consultation times with the GP were all significantly greater for inpatients. Considerable amounts of time were spent by carers looking after their mentally ill relatives, but there was no significant difference between the groups.

Questions

1. Does this study ask an economic question that compares well defined alternative courses of action?   (10 marks)

2. What sort of a study is it? Justify your answer.   (10 marks)

3. Does it cite good evidence on the efficacy of day hospital versus inpatient treatment?   (10 marks)

4. Were all patients randomized to each treatment accounted for at the conclusion of the trial?   (10 marks)

5. How can missing data from one or more subjects be estimated and included in the study calculations?   (20 marks)

6. This study quotes median costs. Why might it do that, and what advantages and disadvantages are there to using it as a measure of cost instead of the mean (list one of each)?

(15 marks)

7. Are the conclusions unlikely to change with sensible changes in costs and outcomes? What sort of analysis is this?

(10 marks)

8. You work in an urban acute mental health unit with access to an acute day unit. You have a large workload of treatment-resistant schizophrenic patients many of whom have had contact with forensic service and are managed in terms of the Mental Health Act. How applicable do you think this study is to your practice? (5 marks)

9. The applicability of a study to other situations is generally influenced by a number of factors. Name two. (10 marks)

Answers

1. Yes. This study compares the effectiveness of day versus inpatient treatment for psychiatric illnesses where admission is avoidable (5 marks). The unit of healthcare improvement is scores on the Comprehensive Psychopathological Rating Scale or the social behaviour checklist (5 marks).

2. It is a cost-effectiveness analysis, based on the result of an RCT (5 marks), as it compares treatments on a cost per unit healthcare improvement (5 marks). The unit of healthcare improvement is the same for both 'therapies'.

3. The economic study is conducted alongside a randomized controlled trial that does not blind clinicians, investigators or patients to which treatment is being received (5 marks). A large double-blind randomized controlled trial would provide a more accurate estimate of treatment effect under ideal conditions (grade Ib evidence) (5 marks).

4. No! Patients assessed with both rating scales seem to be unaccounted for progressively at each time point (5 marks). This may have important implications for the validity of the study, in that to avoid bias dropouts need to be regarded as probable treatment failures (5 marks).

5. Missing data can be handled in a number of different ways. It can be assumed that dropouts can be analysed in the groups to which they were originally randomized. This is the safest method and is called intention-to-treat analysis (5 marks). Missing values can be calculated from the last observation carried forward (5 marks), from the mean of the other members of the group (5 marks), or a treatment failure can be assumed where a dichotomous outcome is measured (5 marks). The last of these is probably based on the safest theoretical assumptions.

6. Median values are less influenced by outliers or from skewness in the shape of a distribution (5 marks). In either of these cases they are more representative of a typical value than the mean (5 marks). However, a mean value can be multiplied by the number of people to obtain a total cost. This is not possible with a median value (5 marks).

7. The name given to an investigation of this sort is a sensitivity analysis (5 marks). It was not conducted in the abstract shown, and therefore we cannot assume that the conclusions are robust to sensible variations in the cost and consequences of therapy (5 marks).

8. The patients in your practice are unlike those of the primary study. Namely, they are largely treatment resistant, have a forensic history, and are generally detained. These were not features of the primary study and are severe limitations to its application to your own practice (5 marks).

9. The applicability of a study is influenced by:
   • Environment of primary study
   • Validity of study
   • Characteristics of participants
   • Inclusion and exclusion criteria
   • Similarity to circumstances of 'real life' (10 marks for any two).

GUIDELINES I

Read the following excerpt from the Bethlem and Maudsley NHS Trust Prescribing Guidelines (Taylor et al 1999) carefully and answer the questions at the end. You may find it easier to read the questions first.

Précis

Algorithm for the drug treatment of schizophrenia

Notes, written at left of algorithm in the primary text:

1. Non-adherence is common, especially if patients do not collaborate in their choice of treatment.

2. Use benzodiazepines or promethazine if sedation or behavioural control is required. Short-term use only (less than 4–6 weeks).

3. Assess drug efficacy with recognized rating scales, e.g. BPRS, CGI.

4. Consider augmentation strategies, e.g. lithium for schizoaffective disorder; carbamazepine for aggression; valproate for mood disturbance.

5. Consider compliance therapy as alternative to depot medication.

6. 'Unproven therapies' if used, must be carefully evaluated using recognized rating scales over a prospectively fixed period (suggest 6–8 weeks). If possible, gain patient consent and document in notes.

Notes on schizophrenia algorithm, written at end of table in the primary text:

1. The algorithm represents an ideal, evidence-based approach to the treatment of schizophrenia and related psychoses.

2. It is assumed that no financial constraints influence drug choice. Where funding is capped or where the use of atypical antipsychotics is restricted to a fixed number of patients, the use of atypicals as first-line may be inappropriate.

3. Low-dose typical antipsychotics may be used first-line where financial restrictions apply. For example, haloperidol 2–4 mg/day can be an effective, well-tolerated regimen. Ideally, atypicals are preferred because of their proven low incidence of extrapyramidal adverse effects, their lack of effect on serum prolactin (not amisulpride or risperidone), and their superior activity against negative symptoms.

4. There is no firm evidence that any drug except clozapine is effective in refractory schizophrenia. Clozapine should be used where two antipsychotics have failed (not more). Note that the longer the duration of poorly treated illness, the worse the prognosis.

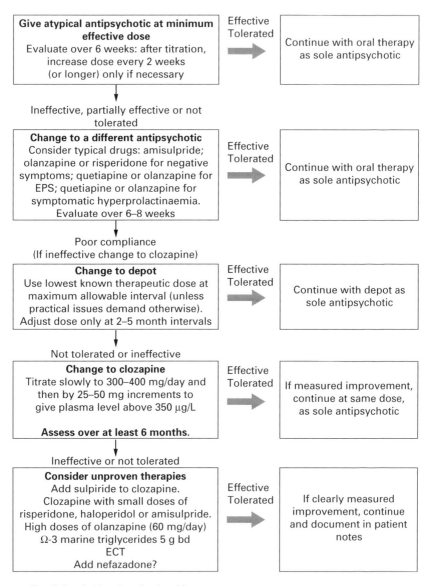

Fig. 5.3 Schizophrenia algorithm

A list of 15 references was given in a later chapter entitled Key References, although they were not cited in the text.

Questions

1. Were all the potentially important treatment options clearly specified? Why is this important? (10 marks)

2. Was all the evidence relevant to each decision option identified, validated and combined in a sensible and explicit way? (15 marks)

3. Is the guideline resistant to clinically sensible variations in practice? (10 marks)

4. How might the guideline affect current clinical practice in your area? (25 marks)

5. What challenges might there be to implementation in your local area and how might these be overcome? (20 marks)

6. Describe the relationship between systematic reviews, meta-analyses, clinical guidelines and clinical audit. (20 marks)

Answers

1. Most pharmacological treatment options are considered, although psychological ones are not (5 marks). All classes of antipsychotic medication are considered, although 'atypicals' are clearly favoured (5 marks).

2. The evidence relevant to each decision is not identified (5 marks), although a list of references is given in the appendix. No explicit consideration is given to the validity of the research and evidence is not graded according to quality and/or precision (5 marks). It is therefore highly uncertain whether it has been combined in a sensible way (5 marks).

3. The guideline covers most variations in clinical practice. It does not take account of psychological therapies, though it does not set out to do this (5 marks). However, the guideline fails to specify the major treatment options and potential outcomes in an explicit way to guide a systematic review (5 marks).

4. There is considerable variation in clinical practice in this field (5 marks). Many doctors prefer one antipsychotic to another, and there is no overall plan to guide current clinical practice (5 marks). Implementation of a guideline such as this may

therefore have considerable effects on clinical practice (5 marks). If it were to improve the treatment of patients with schizophrenia, it could ensure that patients across all wards received the best treatment based on the current best evidence (5 marks). However, there are many reasons to be sceptical of this guideline's validity, as well as its clear favouritism of the more expensive atypical antipsychotic drugs, without a clear and explicit consideration of the evidence (5 marks).

5. My local environment is dissimilar to the catchment area of the Maudsley Hospital (adapt locally) (5 marks). Lack of funding (increase funding, pilot guidelines on one ward, calculate likely costs and benefits) (5 marks). Lack of support from medical staff sceptical about the guideline's validity (enlist collaborators, pilot guideline, enlist local exemplar, etc.) (5 marks). Lack of guideline availability/ease of access (increase supplies, publish wallchart, adapt to a more user-friendly format) (5 marks).

6. Systematic reviews aim to undertake a systematic and comprehensive search for all the published material in a given subject area using reliable and explicit criteria (5 marks). The statistical summary of such data weighted for quality and/or precision is called a meta-analysis (5 marks). Clinical guidelines should be based on a reliable review of the literature, preferably from a systematic review or meta-analysis (5 marks). Such evidence-based guidelines are the best basis for an audit of current clinical practice, as they provide the best evidence of how current clinical practice should be provided (5 marks). However, where evidence cannot be identified, consensus guidelines may sometimes be used.

GUIDELINES II

Read the following brief excerpt from an occasional paper published by the Royal College of Psychiatrists (Royal College of Psychiatrists 1998) and answer the questions at the end.

Précis

The 'management of imminent violence' is a guideline developed by clinical psychologists, psychiatrists, mental health nurses, service users and social workers for the management of imminent or potential violence carried out by non-personality disordered patients without a primary diagnosis of substance misuse. Carers of people with mental health problems were also consulted during guideline development. An evidence review team trained in systematic searching and critical appraisal were enlisted in groups of two or three to one of six subject areas. The areas examined were 'physical environment', 'human environment', 'psychological and social interventions', 'restraint and seclusion', 'medication' and 'prediction'. The programme's recommended databases were EMBASE, PsychLit, MEDLINE and the Cochrane Library. A librarian skilled in supporting evidence-based practice worked closely with the research team. Additional papers were identified by reading the references of review articles and by consulting experts. Studies were rated as meta-analysis, randomized controlled trials, controlled trials, cohort or case–control studies, descriptive and qualitative studies. The recommendations were reviewed widely by a number of professional and voluntary organizations. The findings are published in both long and short form (for easy reference), with a grading of the strength of evidence leading to the recommendation.

Questions

1. Were all the important decision options and outcomes clearly specified? What effect might this have? (10 marks)

2. Was the evidence relevant to each decision option identified, validated and combined in a sensible and explicit way?
(15 marks)

3. Are the relative preferences that key stakeholders attach to the outcomes of decisions identified and explicitly considered? Why is this important? (10 marks)

4. Would the guideline be resistant to clinically sensible variations in practice? (5 marks)

5. Under what circumstances does a guideline offer an opportunity for a significant improvement in practice?
(20 marks)

6. Do you think this guideline offers an opportunity for improvement in your own clinical practice? (10 marks)

7. Could this guideline be implemented in your own clinical practice? What barriers might there be? (10 marks)

8. How might you implement a guideline? How might you help ensure its success? (20 marks)

Answers

1. All important decisions and outcomes, based on the précis, do not seem to have been considered explicitly and in depth (5 marks). Therefore, many important interventions and their consequences may have been missed (5 marks).

2. Again, the authors say they have reviewed several subject areas that they specify. However, exact search terms are not specified in a way that would allow the search to be repeated (5 marks). They could also have contacted pharmaceutical companies for unpublished material and performed a hand search to identify more potentially relevant material (5 marks). They say that each article was critically appraised and then graded, according to the type of study. Exactly how this was done is not specified explicitly or in any depth (5 marks).

3. Yes, at the beginning of the guideline the stakeholders are listed and their relevant backgrounds given (5 marks). The guideline canvasses a wide range of different perspectives. The relevant preferences that key stakeholders attach to each outcome are not specified in the précis, but may be specified in the original publication. This is important, because the values and preferences assumed by a guideline must be a good match for the values and preferences of those on whom it will be used (5 marks). Recommendations unacceptable to large numbers of patients will be difficult to implement successfully.

4. The guideline does not consider most options and outcomes explicitly, at least according to the précis. It is therefore uncertain whether it would be resistant to sensible variations in clinical practice. The guideline excludes those with a primary diagnosis of substance misuse or personality disorder, a potentially violent group in routine clinical practice whose management would not be usefully aided by the adoption of this guideline (5 marks).

5. A guideline offers significant opportunity for improvements in practice where there is a large variation in clinical practice (5

marks), there is the potential to spend resources more effectively (opportunity costs) (5 marks), or where it is possible to improve the treatment of a large number of individuals at low risk (5 marks) or a smaller number of individuals at high risk (5 marks).

6. Yes. I know that clinical practice in psychiatry varies somewhat. Furthermore, the patients seen by general adult psychiatry tend to be at the severe end of the clinical spectrum, therefore if their care was enhanced significantly a considerable improvement in outcome could result (10 marks for any reasoned justification). However, the concerns about the validity of the guideline may mean that it does not apply to many violent situations commonly encountered in routine clinical practice.

7. (a) Lack of willingness by clinicians, managers, pharmacists, nurses, etc.
   (b) Lack of similarity to environment of guideline
   (c) Lack of funds
   (d) Lack of availability (10 marks for all four correct, or 2 marks each).

8. (a) Enlist key colleagues and local exemplars
   (b) Pilot on your own ward
   (c) Adapt locally
   (d) Supply in user-friendly format
   (e) Enlist colleagues at the development stage
   (f) Opportunity for individual discussion with a respected authority
   (g) Try to ensure it is free from conflict with economic and administrative perspectives and patient and community perspectives (20 marks for any 5, or 4 marks each).

AUDIT I

Read the précis from a published paper in the *British Journal of Psychiatry* (Donoghue & Tylee 1996) and answer the questions at the end.

Précis

Information on antidepressant prescribing by GPs was obtained from three independent data sources. Prescribing analysis and cost (PACT) provided information on the number of prescriptions written for each strength of antidepressants prescribed during the first quarter of 1993. Information on doses was approximated from this on the assumption that GPs usually prescribe in cycles of 1 month, and that all these were for depression. Three GPs gave permission to access the notes of those patients who were on antidepressants in the past 12 months. DIN-LINK computerized database maintains data from GPs in 100 practices and uses the AAH-MEDITEL practice computer. Daily dose and quantity of medication were collected for all patients diagnosed as having depression over the same period as the PACT data. Consensus guidelines issued by the Royal College of Psychiatrists and General Practitioners on the treatment of depression in primary care and those by the British Association of Psychopharmacology were used for recommendations on effective doses. χ^2 analyses were done to compare differences between older and newer antidepressants in terms of the number of prescriptions which reached effective doses.

The results are given in Table 5.13.

Table 5.13   Percentage of antidepressant prescriptions at effective dose measured by three independent data sources

	Older TCA % effective dose	Lofepramine % effective dose	SSRI % effective dose	P value
PACT	13.4	61.4	98.1	<0.001
DIN-LINK	12.04	78.83	99.26	<0.001
GP notes	25	95	100	<0.001

TCA = tricyclic antidepressants; SSRI = specific serotonin reuptake inhibitors.

Questions

1. What were reference guidelines for doing this audit? Explain how a good guideline should be generated. Are consensus guidelines valid?   (15 marks)

2. What were the various ways in which data were collected? Can you rank these in order of quality of their reliability, giving reasons for each? Can you name the major disadvantage of each source as you rank?   (15 marks)

3. The authors note that the prescription of SSRIs was more likely to be in the therapeutic range: can you explain why? Give two reasons. (10 marks)

4. Expert guidelines are based on treatment trials. How does this compare with the patients seen in primary care? (15 marks)

5. What was missing in the results for you to make a definite conclusion that the GPs' treatment of depression was inadequate? (5 marks)

6. What kind of audit will truly answer whether the treatment of depression in primary care is effective or not? (15 marks)

7. Describe the components of an audit cycle. (10 marks)

8. Explain how the results of this audit can be used to improve services. (15 marks)

Answers

1. Consensus guidelines of the Royal College of Psychiatrists and General Practitioners and Guidelines of the British Association of Psychopharmacology (5 marks for both).

   Generation of guidelines:

   (a) An explicit method should be stated for the selection of research papers needed to generate the guidelines.

   (b) The quality of evidence used to generate these guidelines should be clearly stated, e.g. randomized trials, systematic reviews, etc.

   (c) An objective method should be used for rating the identified papers and compiling the guidelines. (5 marks)

   Consensus guidelines are popular but not valid if there is sufficient material to generate an evidence-based guideline as described above. In the absence of sufficient research consensus guidelines are valid (5 marks).

2. (a) *GP notes*: This gives information on the diagnosis, the antidepressant prescribed, duration of treatment and the dose. However, only three GPs' notes were accessed, therefore the generalizability of data is limited.

   (b) *DIN-LINK database*: This has information on antidepressants and daily dose prescribed. It does not include information on diagnosis and includes only those practices that have a specified computer system.

(c) *PACT data*: Gives information on the number of prescriptions written, the quantity prescribed and the strength. It does not give information on the dose or the diagnosis. A rough approximation is made as to how much each patient may have had as a daily dose.

(5 marks each = 15 marks)

3. The initial dose of almost all SSRIs is within the therapeutic range, whereas all tricyclics need titration up to therapeutic doses. GPs may not be familiar with the titration regimen, or may not know the therapeutic range of doses. GPs may also use low doses of TCAs because of the risk of overdose and toxicity (5 marks for each point to a maximum of 10 marks).

4. Although not mentioned in the paper, expert guidelines are presumably based on randomized controlled trials of patients with depressive disorders (5 marks). Such trials select a strictly defined range of patients usually in contact with secondary care (5 marks). Patients with depression in general practice may be very different from those in the trial population in terms of their course and outcome with treatment (5 marks).

5. The outcome of treatments is not mentioned. Unless information on outcome is available it is hard to assume that the treatments given by GPs were ineffective (5 marks).

6. An audit for these purposes will involve
   - Establishing a diagnosis in all patients started on antidepressants, as different diagnoses may respond to different doses (for example, obsessive–compulsive disorder is treated with higher initial doses of SSRIs than is depression)
   - Making a note of doses and duration of treatment
   - Measuring outcomes objectively

   (5 marks for each point to a maximum of 15 marks)

   The categories in this example are therapeutic or non-therapeutic prescriptions of older versus newer antidepressants.

7. Please include the diagram of the audit cycle. (See Chapter 4 for a diagram of the audit cycle.) (5 marks for two correct entries, 10 marks for all entries correct).

8. The audit results can be used to optimize the prescribing of antidepressants of various classes (5 marks). More attention can be paid to depression in primary care and its treatment, and how this may be different from that in secondary care (5 marks). As depression is a common problem appropriate information should be provided to the GPs regarding its treatment and prognosis (5 marks).

AUDIT II

Read the following précis of a published article (Carr et al 1997), and answer the questions at the end.

Précis

Over a 12-month period 307 referrals were made by GPs to a primary care consultation–liaison psychiatric service: 86 of these agreed to participate in this study of outcome. Out of a representative group of 1280 who had psychiatric symptoms but were not referred to the C–L team, 86 controls were selected. Both sociodemographic and symptom matching were attempted to provide broader comparisons. The selection of study and control groups is outlined below.

Study group selection

305 referrals
259 eligible   46 removed (too young or too unwell)
86 agree
78 agree to interview and questions
7 agree to questions only
1 agrees to interview only

Control group selection

1280
816 agree to be contacted
535 complete questionnaires
86 selected as sociodemographic controls
59 clinically matched   27 not matched symptomatically

Participants underwent composite international diagnostic interview (CIDI) at home by a researcher blind to their group membership. The interview was done 2–4 weeks after GP contact and yielded DSM-III R diagnoses. Questionnaires completed at initial assessment and 6 months later were SCL-90–R symptom checklist; social support; recent life event scale; Eysenck Personality Inventory; and a variety of health and activity related subjective ratings. Table 5.14 summarizes the diagnostic subtypes.

Table 5.14 Diagnosic characteristics of patients referred to a consultation–liaison service and those who were not

Diagnosis	C–L referrals (n = 79)		Controls (n = 76)	
	n	%	n	%
Substance	9	11.4	3	3.9
Mood disorder	30	38	4	5.3
Anxiety disorder	37	46.8	21	21.6
Somatoform disorder	13	16.5	2	2.6
Others	2	2.5	2	2.6
None	13	16.5	52	68.4

C–L referrals were younger, commonly female, and more likely to be single, unemployed or students and of lower socioeconomic status. There was 59% agreement between CIDI and clinical diagnosis. ANOVA showed a significant main effect for symptom severity in the 74 C–L subjects (who had completed follow-up) compared with the 76 demographic controls. The C–L subjects had more severe symptoms. Although symptoms improved over time in both the groups, there was no group by time interaction for symptom profile. There were no differences between symptom matched C–L referrals and controls on any of the outcome variables.

Questions

1. What is the purpose of clinical audits? (5 marks)

2. Is the sample representative of the patients referred to liaison services? Support your answer with two arguments. (15 marks)

3. Give two reasons why there was a high proportion of females in the referred group. (10 marks)

4. What could be the reasons for disagreement between CIDI and clinical diagnosis? (10 marks)

5. In what manner was the control limb of the audit designed? How do the investigators justify two control groups? (15 marks)

6. A statistical technique called ANOVA has been used in this paper. Explain its utility. What do the terms main effects and interaction mean with respect to ANOVA technique?

(25 marks)

7. What could be the reason for lack of any significant difference in the objective outcome of the three groups?

(10 marks)

8. Would you be in favour of a C–L primary care team in your set up? Explain with reference to this paper. (10 marks)

Answers

1. A clinical audit is research aimed at studying the processes of a healthcare activity (5 marks).

2. The sample is not representative of the patients referred to the primary care psychiatric liaison services (5 marks).
   (a) Out of the total 305 of referrals only 86 eventually agreed to participate.
   (b) The very ill patients were not included in the analysis. (5 marks each = 10 marks).

3. (a) After the severe mental disorders were excluded the sample consisted of chiefly anxiety and mood disorders. These have a higher incidence in the female sex.
   (b) Females may have been seen as more vulnerable and needing extra help. (5 marks each = 10 marks)

4. (a) Clinicians were GPs and they may not have a high expertise in psychiatric diagnoses.
   (b) The CIDI interview was done at a different time and place (patients' homes) from the clinical interview. The symptom picture may have changed. (5 marks each = 10 marks)

5. The investigators tried to match as many patients in the study group with the control group for sociodemographic and symptomatic variables. However, only 59 could be so matched. The rest (27) were matched based on socio-demographic details only. The investigators claim that this

would give them answers based on patients' symptoms and background. (5 marks each = 15 marks)

6. ANOVA stands for analysis of variance (5 marks). This test is used to compare continuous or interval scores of more than two groups (5 marks). In this example we have scores from the study group and two control groups (5 marks). Effect refers to a statistical difference that is the result of the influence of one variable (5 marks). Interaction refers to the combined influence of two variables to produce a difference between groups (5 marks).

7. The severely ill are more likely to improve but have not been included in the study (5 marks). Those who are included probably have milder symptoms, which easily reach a ceiling for improvement no matter how they are treated (5 marks). The follow-up of 6 months may not be enough to compare differences in outcome (5 marks—any two of the three accepted).

8. A C–L team will not be useful for all or even most patients with psychiatric problems in primary care, as shown in this paper (5 marks). Patients who are more severely ill may benefit. Therefore, a liaison with commitment to this small group may be most effective (5 marks).

REFERENCES AND FURTHER READING

Brown T, Wilkinson G 1998 Critical Reviews in Psychiatry. London: Gaskell (Royal College of Psychiatrists)

Carr VJ, Lewin TJ, Reid ALA, Walton JM, Faehrmann C 1997 Evaluation of effectiveness of consultation–liaison psychiatry service in the general practice. Australian and New Zealand Journal of Psychiatry 31: 714–725

Creed F, Mbaya P, Lancashire S, Tomenson B, Williams B, Holme S 1997 Cost effectiveness of day and inpatient psychiatric treatment: results of a randomised controlled trial. British Medical Journal 314: 1381–1385

Donoghue JM, Tylee A 1996 The treatment of depression: prescribing patterns of antidepressants in primary care in the UK. British Journal of Psychiatry 168: 164–168

Duggan C, Sham P, Minnie C, Lee A, Murray R 1998 Family history as a predictor of poor long-term outcome of depression. British Journal of Psychiatry 173: 527–536

Elliot AJ, Uldall KK, Bergman K, Russo J, Claypoole K, Roy-Byrne PP 1998 Randomized, placebo-controlled trial of paroxetine versus imipramine in depressed HIV-positive outpatients. American Journal of Psychiatry 155: 367–372

Hulse GK, Milne E, English DR, Holman CDJ 1998 Assessing the relationship between maternal opiate use and neonatal mortality. Addiction 93: 1033–1042

Klein E, Kreinin I, Chistyakov A et al 1999 Therapeutic efficacy of right prefrontal slow repetitive transcranial magnetic stimulation in major depression: a double-blind controlled study. Archives of General Psychiatry 56: 315–320

Kraft MK, Rothbard AB, Hadley TR, McLellan AT, Asch DA 1998 Are supplementary services provided during methadone maintenance really cost-effective? American Journal of Psychiatry 154: 1214–1219

Morgan JF, Reid F, Lacey JH 1999 The SCOFF questionaire: assessment of a new screening tool for eating disorders. British Medical Journal 319: 1467–1468

O'Brien BJ, Ames D, Chiu E, Schweitzer I, Desmond P, Tess B 1998 Severe deep white matter lesions and outcome in elderly patients with major depressive disorder: follow up study. British Medical Journal 317: 982–984

Royal College of Psychiatrists (1998) Management of imminent violence; clinical practice guidlines to support mental health services. Royal College of Psychiatrists, London

Sadowski H, Ugarte B, Kolvin I, Kaplan C, Barnes J 1999 Early life family disadvantage and major depression in adulthood. British Journal of Psychiatry 174: 112–120

Taylor D, McConnell D, McConnell H, Abel K, Kerwin R 1999 Treatment of psychosis. In: The Bethlem and Maudsley NHS Trust prescribing guidelines, 5th edn. London: Martin Dunitz, 21–37

van Os J, Selten JP 1998 Prenatal exposure to maternal stress and subsequent schizophrenia. The May 1940 invasion of the Netherlands. British Journal of Psychiatry 172: 324–326

Glossary

Absolute benefit increase (ABI): the absolute numerical difference between the rates of good outcomes between experimental and control participants in a trial.

Absolute risk reduction (ARR): the absolute numerical difference between the rates of adverse outcomes in the control and experimental groups.

Alpha (α): the probability of a type I error.

Analysis of variance (ANOVA): a statistical test where three or more groups are compared on a single continuous measure. The groups must be independent and the data normally distributed and at least interval.

Beta (β): the probability of falsely accepting the null hypothesis (i.e. the probability of demonstrating no difference, where in fact a true difference exists).

Bias: processes leading to the systematic deviation of results from the truth.

Binomial distribution: a specific statistical distribution of a discrete random variable. Used for hypothesis testing where proportions are involved, e.g. the 95%CI for a prognosis study.

Blinding: a term used in randomized controlled trials (RCTs). Single blinding is where patients are unaware of the intervention received. Double-blind studies are where neither clinician nor patient is aware of the intervention received. Triple blinding is where outcome raters are also blind.

Case–control study: a generally retrospective study of two or more groups of people defined by the presence of an outcome or disease.

Case series: a report on a series of patients with an outcome of interest. There is no control group.

Ceiling effect: a term used when the values of many subjects on a variable are near the maximum possible value 'ceiling'. This causes a problem for certain types of analysis because it reduces the possible variation in the sample. Where values are near the minimum possible limit, the term 'floor' effect is used.

Central limit theorem: a statement that as the sample size increases, the sample mean will approach a normal distribution, no matter what the shape of the parent population is. Relevant to the interpretation of the standard error.

Chi-square (χ^2) test: a non-parametric statistical test that compares expected frequencies with observed frequencies of categorical data.

Clinical effectiveness: see Effectiveness.

Clinical practice guideline: a systematically developed statement designed to assist clinicians and patients make decisions about important healthcare options in specific circumstances.

Cluster analysis: a technique that aims to separate complex data sets into homogeneous categories.

Cochrane Collaboration: an international venture to systematically find, appraise and review available evidence from RCTs.

Cochrane Library: a regularly updated electronic library of evidence from the Cochrane Collaboration comprising the Cochrane Database of Systematic Reviews (CDSR), the Database of Abstracts of Reviews of Effectiveness (DARE), the Cochrane Controlled Trials Register (CCTR) and the Cochrane Review Methodology Database (CRMD).

Cohort study: a generally prospective epidemiological study of one or more groups, defined by the presence or absence of an exposure (aetiology study) or a disease (prognosis study).

Confidence interval (95%): the range of values in which we can be 95% confident that the true value of a given population parameter lies.

Confounder: a variable associated with both exposure and outcome but not on the causal pathway.

Control event rate: the proportion of people in the control (non-exposed) group of a clinical trial who experience a specified event.

Correlation: a measure of the degree of association between two or more variables. Correlation coefficients range from -1 to $+1$.

Cost–benefit analysis: an economic analysis that compares the costs and outcomes of two or more therapeutic manoeuvres in terms of monetary value.

Cost-effectiveness study: an economic analysis that compares two or more treatments in terms of the cost per unit healthcare gain.

Cost–utility analysis: an economic analysis that compares two or more treatments in terms of the cost per quality-adjusted life year gained.

Cronbach's α: an index of the internal consistency of a test.

Crossover study: the administration of two or more experimental treatments after each other to the same group of patients in a clinical trial.

Cross-sectional study: a study where information is collected from a given population at a specific time point.

Degrees of freedom (df): an elusive concept. It is essentially a measure of the numbers of ways in which a data set may vary. Usually given by $n-1$.

Descriptive statistics: methods of summarizing data. Includes mean, median, mode and standard deviation.

Discrete variable: variables that have only integer values.

Discriminant analysis: a technique that allows individuals to be separated into different groups according to a given rule or function.

Ecological fallacy: a spurious association found in an ecological study between an exposure and an outcome at a population level that does not hold at an individual level.

Ecological study: a study based on aggregated data from a given population designed to investigate the relationship between an exposure and an outcome.

Effectiveness: the beneficial effects of a manoeuvre under clinical (real-life) conditions.

Efficacy: the beneficial effects of a manoeuvre under experimental conditions.

Efficiency: the effects achieved in relation to the effort expended in terms of money, resources and time.

Event rate: the proportion of patients in whom a given event is observed over a given time period.

Evidence-based medicine: the conscientious, explicit and judicious use of the current best evidence in making decisions about the care of individual patients.

Experimental event rate: the proportion of people in the experimental (exposed) group who experience a specified event.

Exposure: an epidemiological term for any factor that is associated with an outcome and may therefore be causal.

Factor analysis: a name given to a group of statistical techniques that aim to reduce large complex data sets to a smaller number of explanatory variables.

Factorial analysis of variance: a statistical test that compares the mean of a dependent measure when the sample can be classified in different ways, e.g. sex, treatment group, diagnosis, etc.

Fisher's exact probability test: an alternative to the χ^2 test when the frequencies of each event are small.

Fixed effects analysis: a method used in meta-analysis where two or more studies are combined and there is low heterogeneity.

F test: a test for the equality of variances of two populations, given by the ratio of the between-groups variance to the within-group variance. Most often calculated using the analysis of variance (ANOVA).

Galbraith plot: a plot of the standard normal deviate against the reciprocal of the standard error. Used to investigate heterogeneity but can be adapted to study and quantify publication bias.

Halo effect: the tendency of a rater to overestimate a subject's response based on prior assumptions.

Hawthorne effect: the non-specific effects caused by the knowledge subjects have that they are participating in an experimental study. The term originates from the Hawthorne Plant in Chicago.

Heterogeneity: a term used in meta-analysis where several studies' results differ more than would be expected by chance.

Histogram: a graphical representation of data whereby the class interval is represented upon the x-axis (abscissa) and the frequencies are represented in the area of each rectangle.

Hotellings T^2: a test statistic used with multivariate analysis of variance. Other tests include Wilk's λ.

Hypothesis testing: used to asses whether experimental data are consistent with prior statements made about the population from which they were drawn.

Incidence: the proportion of new events in a population at risk in a specified time period (incidence risk) or in a certain number of person-years of observation (incidence rate).

Incremental analysis: a term used in health economics that examines the additional costs that one service or programme imposes over another, compared with the additional effects, benefits or utilities it delivers.

Intention-to-treat analysis: a method whereby the data produced in the course of a clinical trial are analysed according to the group patients were originally randomized to.

Interval scale: a measurement scale where there is an equal interval between the units of measurement.

Kappa (κ): a measure of diagnostic agreement corrected for agreement expected by chance.

Kruskal–Wallis test: a non-parametric (distribution-free) statistical test that compares the median (or mean rank) of three or more groups. Sometimes called a Kruskal–Wallis ANOVA.

Kurtosis: a measure of how far data depart from the standard normal distribution around the mean. Data may be more flattened (platykurtic) or more peaked (leptokurtic).

Last observation carried forward: a type of analysis used to estimate a missing value in a clinical trial from the last measurement in an individual subject.

Likelihood ratio: the value of a given test result in predicting the presence of disease. Numerically, this is the probability of a test result in diseased individuals divided by the probability of the same result in control subjects.

Likert scale: a scale where a subject is asked to respond to a question by marking one of a series of *discrete* points on a dimension.

Mann–Whitney U test: a statistical test that compares the ranks of values of two groups.

McNemar's test: a test for comparing observed and expected frequencies of paired data.

Mean: the average value obtained by adding all measurements together and dividing by the total number of measurements.

Median: the average value that divides the distribution into two equal parts. The middle value.

Meta-analysis: a combination of two or more studies weighted for quality and/or precision.

Mode: the value that occurs most frequently in a data set.

Multiple regression: a form of regression where one determines the best combination of independent variables to predict a dependent variable.

Multivariate analysis of variance (MANOVA): a statistical test that compares two or more independent groups on two or more dependent measures.

Negative predictive value (NPV): the proportion of people who score negative in a test who actually do not have the disorder.

Nominal scale: a measurement scale where numbers are used to represent categories but have no rank order.

Non-parametric statistics: statistical techniques that do not rely upon normally distributed continuous data with (approximately) equal variances.

Null hypothesis: a statement that there is no difference, or no association, between two or more groups in a study.

Number needed to harm: the number of patients who, if they receive the experimental treatment, would lead to one additional person being harmed, compared with patients who receive the control treatment.

Number needed to treat: the inverse of the absolute risk reduction, and is the number of patients that need to be treated to prevent one bad outcome compared with a control treatment.

Odds: the ratio of probabilities of an event happening to its not happening. If the probability for a disease is 0.1 (10%), the probability of the disease not happening is 0.9 and therefore its odds are 9:1.

Odds ratio: compares the odds of an event happening in one group to that of it happening in another group. The two groups could be experimental and control groups as in treatment studies, or exposed and not-exposed groups as in case-control studies.

Ordinal scale: a level of measurement where numbers refer to the rank order of variables, but where the intervals between numbers are not equal (e.g. social class).

Overview: is a (systematic) review and summary of the (medical) literature.

Paired tests: statistical tests used in paired samples where each observation in a data set has one matching observation in another.

Parametric statistics: those statistical techniques that rely upon assumptions such as independence, equal variance, at least interval or continuous data and normal distribution.

Patient expected event rate (PEER): refers to the rate of events expected in patients who received no treatment or conventional treatment in the setting of the clinical practice in question.

Pearson's correlation coefficient: a correlation coefficient between two normally distributed continuous variables.

Positive predictive value (PPV): the proportion of people who score positive in a test who actually have the disorder.

Power (1 − β): the probability of demonstrating a significant difference between groups where one exists. Also equal to the probability of not making a type II error.

Pretest odds: the odds that a patient has a disorder before the diagnostic test is carried out.

Pretest probability/prevalence: the proportion of people with the target disorder in a population at risk at a specific time point or interval.

Prevalence: the proportion of people in a sample who have the disorder, measured generally with a diagnostic gold standard.

***P* value**: the probability that the observed results of a study could have occurred by chance. The probability of falsely rejecting the null hypothesis.

Proportion: a type of ratio in which the numerator is included in the denominator. The ratio of a part to a whole expressed as a decimal fraction. Must lie between 0 and 1.

Randomized controlled trial: a controlled trial in which a group of patients is randomized into an experimental group and a control group.

Rate: a ratio whose essential characteristic is that time is an element of the denominator. However, the term is also used less strictly to refer to a proportion.

Ratio: the value obtained by dividing one quantity by another. It differs from a proportion, in which the numerator is included in the population defined by the denominator; this is not necessarily the case with a ratio.

Ratio scale: a measurement scale where the units are equally spaced, there is an inherent order, and a true zero exists.

Recall bias: bias introduced by the selective memory of subjects or informants.

Receiver operating characteristic (ROC) curve: a graphical means for assessing the ability of a diagnostic test to discriminate between healthy and diseased individuals. Originally a term used in psychometry, where the characteristic operating response of a individual to faint stimuli or non-stimuli was recorded.

Regression: closely related to correlation, regression is the prediction of a dependent variable based on its relationship with another, independent variable.

Regression to the mean: the tendency for extreme values on a measure to decrease with repeated measurement or time. For example, if a group of high scoring individuals is followed up over time, it is usual to find their scores have reduced at retesting.

Relative benefit increase: the RBI is the increase in rates of good events, comparing experimental and control patients in a trial, as a ratio to the event rate in controls.

Relative risk increase: the RRI is the increase in rates of bad events, comparing the experimental patients with control patients in a trial, as a ratio to the event rate in controls.

Relative risk reduction: relative risk reduction is the percent reduction in events in experimental group (EER) compared with controls (CER) or (CER-EER)/CER.

Response bias: bias introduced by the selective response or non-response of particular subjects.

Risk ratio the ratio of risk in the treated group (EER) to that in the control group (CER) – used in randomized trials and cohort studies.

Scheffé (post hoc) test: a post hoc test used most commonly with an analysis of variance to detect where significant differences lie.

Sensitivity: the proportion of people who truly have the disorder who are detected as positive by the particular test.

Sensitivity analysis: a statistical technique used to examine uncertainties about a study's conclusions.

Skewness: a departure from the normal distribution, where either the 'left' or the 'right' hand tail of the distribution is longer than would be expected. Positive skew is where the right-hand tail is extended and the mean>median>mode. Negative skew extends the left hand tail and mode>median>mean. Generally the mean is most affected by skew.

Specificity: the proportion of people who do not have the disorder who are classed as negative by the particular test.

Standard deviation (SD): a standardized measure of data dispersion. Calculated as

$$\frac{\sum (x-\bar{x})^2}{(n-1)} \quad \text{(sample standard deviation)}.$$

Standard error (SE): a measure of the uncertainty, or dispersion, of a point estimate such as the sample mean. Used to construct confidence intervals and calculated as

$$\frac{SD}{\sqrt{n}}$$

Statistic: a numerical characteristic of a sample.

Statistical significance: a result highly unlikely to have occurred by chance alone.

Systematic review: a review of research papers, selected using prespecified criteria.

Transformation: a change in the scale of a measurement by a mathematical function. Commonly used functions include square root, log and inverse. Usually used so that data are normally distributed and parametric statistical methods can be used.

t **test**: a parametric test for the difference between two means.

Two-tailed test: a test that there is a significant difference between two measurements or values in either direction (greater or smaller).

Type I error: the false rejection of the null hypothesis where no true difference exists.

Type II error: the false acceptance of the null hypothesis where a true difference exists.

Utility: a health state preference score.

Wilcoxon's signed rank test: a non-parametric (distribution-free) test for measuring the difference between two paired samples.

Variance: a standardized measure of data dispersion. Equal to the standard deviation squared.

z **score**: a data transformation calculated by subtracting the mean from every value and dividing by the standard deviation. The transformed scores have useful properties and are assumed to follow the standard normal distribution, with mean 0 and a standard deviation of 1.

Index

261